"This is an unusually moving and inspirational book, a clear-eyed and loving portrait of a son and his too-short but transcendent life. Graham's story is a tribute to the human spirit and the invisible bonds which connect us to each other."

—Ken Burns, Documentary Filmmaker

"The story of a beautiful boy who showed us a life without limits and embodied the power of love."

—Katie Couric, Journalist

"To what lengths would the loving parents of a severely disabled child go to enrich his life? And in return, what profound lessons would that child teach all who nurtured him? Readers of *Jabberwocky* will be pondering those questions long after they finish this remarkable story."

—Joseph P. Kahn, columnist, Boston Globe

"How lucky we are that Steven and Cynthia were chosen to receive the gift of Graham and that they knew he was meant to be shared. In Graham's world-including a madcap summer camp called Jabberwocky-something wondrous and beyond us is at play..."

—Robin Young, NPR host

"This is a holy book."

—Rabbi Lawrence Kushner

"It was a story I needed to hear. It was a deeply spiritual story. Graham reflected beauty, goodness, and humility into a self-absorbed, goal-driven, power-hungry world. For those who were present and aware, Graham taught them life changing lessons of life. And his spirit continues to do so!"

—Phil Reppert, author of *Nativity on East 7th,*
a New York City Christmas Love Story

"Graham Gardner was an example of the invaluable place in this world that is occupied by people who are "greatly different." And no boy was ever more beloved by his father, in a world that aches for fathers who love their sons."

—Dr. Gina Higgins, psychologist and author
of *Resilient Adults: Overcoming a Cruel Past*

JABBERWOCKY

JABBERWOCKY

LESSONS OF LOVE FROM
A BOY WHO NEVER SPOKE

DR. STEVEN GARDNER

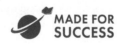

MADE FOR
SUCCESS

Made for Success Publishing
P.O. Box 1775 Issaquah, WA 98027
www.MadeForSuccessPublishing.com

Distributed by Made for Success Publishing

First Printing

Library of Congress Cataloging-in-Publication data
Gardner, Dr. Steven
    JABBERWOCKY: Lessons of Love from a Boy Who Never Spoke
        p. cm.

    LCCN: 2021934741
    ISBN: 978-1-64146-624-0 (*Hardback*)
    ISBN: 978-1-64146-630-1 (*eBook*)
    ISBN: 978-1-64146-647-9 (*Audiobook*)

Printed in the United States of America

For further information contact Made for Success Publishing

+14255266480 or email service@madeforsuccess.net

"Grief is the price we pay for love."
—Queen Elizabeth II

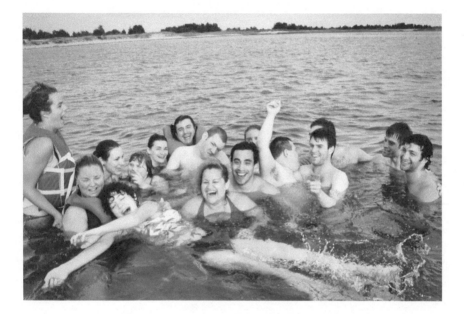

*This book is dedicated
to the people of Camp Jabberwocky,
past, present, and future.*

Contents

Foreword

Come to my arms, my beamish boy!
O frabjous day! Callooh! Callay!
He chortled in his joy.

"Jabberwocky"
Lewis Carroll

Farewell, thou child of my right hand and joy;
My sin was too much hope of thee, loved boy.

"On My First Son"
Ben Jonson

For 150 years, "Jabberwocky" has been an iconic, magical poem. But, for more than 65 years, Jabberwocky has been an iconic, magical camp on Martha's Vineyard for severely disabled adults and children. It's a joyous place where campers and the counselors who must care for them every minute are the happiest people on an island populated by the prosperous, powerful, and privileged—who are reminded by Jabberwocky of how fortunate they are and how grateful they should be. Jabberwocky is also now an inspired and inspiring book about the profound bond between Graham Gardner, a boy with severe cerebral palsy, and his father, Steven, a doctor who ultimately could not save his beloved son.

This is not a sad story. It is filled with the madcap adventures of Jabberwocky counselors and their campers, who, for a short time each summer, are not limited by their disabilities and raucously soar.

It is the story of Graham, so intensely loved by Steven (and his mother Cynthia) that he radiated kindness, brought out the very best in everyone he met and became widely known as an "Angel in Service of God."

No father would wish for a severely disabled son—a son who would never walk, talk, or play catch. Yet Steven's devotion to meeting Graham's demanding needs and creating unlikely shared experiences—including kayaking, windsurfing, swimming, and skiing—forged an intimacy that inspires envy, not pity.

Jabberwocky is funny. *Jabberwocky* is joyful. *Jabberwocky* is poignant. *Jabberwocky* is also important. It prompts us to pause and think deeply about what gives meaning to life and how to live it.

Lord Byron wrote that "There is no joy the world can give like that it takes away." However, *Jabberwocky* is a reminder that, as Mitch Albom wrote in *Tuesdays with Morrie,* while death ends a life, it does not end a relationship. Despite the excruciating pain of losing the living Graham, *Jabberwocky* is a testament to the love of a father for his son that will never die, and to a joy that will never end.

We are fortunate to have *Jabberwocky*—another of Graham's great gifts.

—The Honorable Mark L. Wolf, Senior United States District Judge

Prologue

Dear Bud,

The world went on, as it always does when someone leaves it, but it was a far more wonderful place with you in it. Even all these words—71,000 of them—cannot adequately express how it felt to be your father. Or how it feels now to go on living without you.

Inevitably, the memories of a lifetime fade with time, even the rare, singularly thrilling ones. But I don't want to ever forget the details of our life together. With you here, your mother and I experienced the transformative power of loving absolutely and being loved absolutely in return. We came to understand the true feeling of joy. And, with you around, life was whimsical and fun—in so many unexpected ways.

As your mom memorably said, being around Graham Gardner was "like having the sun shine on your whole being." Now, that magical aura no longer envelops us.

"There was a kind of nobility in your life when you were with Graham," said one friend. Quite right. Not too many people are given the chance to know that feeling—how lucky we were to experience that gift from you.

Proud is not a strong enough word for how you made us feel.

So, what now, for those of us left behind?

We can try to pay forward some of the kindness you embodied. We can remind ourselves to persevere, even when life is painful, because that is what you did so often. We can treat people who are different from us respectfully, as you did.

And above all, we can try to be loving, as you were so abundantly, every day of your life.

At the same time, Bud, we can hope, with all our hearts, that when our own time comes to "cross over," we will have the chance to embrace you once again.

When you were a baby I wrote a lullaby for you with this refrain:

> "*I am yours and you are mine*
> *And we are parts of one design*
> *Like branches on a tree*
> *Waves out on the sea*
> *Notes sung in two-part harmony*
> *And all I really want to do*
> *Is share*
> *This life with you.*"

Until we meet again my beautiful boy,

All my love,

Dad

AT FIRST

Nothing seemed strange at the beginning. Cynthia and I were first-time parents. We knew little about the developmental milestones that babies are expected to reach at certain dates during the first year of life. We had a beautiful baby boy who was unusually cranky. That was all. But, at some indiscernible point in time, Cynthia and I developed concerns. They were vague at first.

Our gorgeous son, Graham, would not hold a rattle. He did not try to crawl, and he would not follow a moving object, like his mother's face, with his eyes. He rarely slept and appeared uncomfortable much of the time. The pediatrician found nothing obviously wrong except that his head circumference was very small, according to the growth charts in the exam room. On subsequent visits, we watched with increasing trepidation as the physician connected the dots on those simple graphs. The routine ritual of the "well-baby visit" became a source of dread. Graham's head circumference was not catching up with even the lowest of the normal growth curves, suggesting that his brain was not developing properly.

On a sultry July day, while I was holding him in our little yard in the seaside town of Marblehead, fifteen miles north of Boston, Graham had a grand mal seizure. A kindly neighbor who was watering her garden across the street drove us to the local ER so that we would not have to wait for an ambulance. The convulsion continued during the harrowing ride to the hospital as I held our tiny child against my chest, trying frantically to keep him from biting his tongue.

I was an internal medicine physician on the staff of that very hospital, and I had seen every kind of medical emergency during my residency training at Boston's Massachusetts General Hospital (MGH). But the sight of my own son, unconscious and flailing wildly, being stuck with needles in order to administer intravenous medicines, was horrifying. I watched in panic as the IV drug that finally stopped Graham's seizure also stopped his breathing. The pediatric resident and I frantically grabbed a tiny bag valve mask and pushed air into Graham's lungs. Luck was with us in the form of a senior anesthesiologist who happened to be in the ER that weekend day. The calm gray-haired stranger quietly took over and skillfully "bagged" Graham with oxygen from the device for nearly an hour before I saw my son finally start to breathe on his own.

After that day, Cynthia and I faced the possibility that something was seriously wrong with our son. Following a dizzying series of tests and specialist visits, we asked for a meeting with Graham's pediatrician. For the first time, we heard the term *cerebral palsy* (CP) applied to our boy. The doctor hadn't wanted to have that conversation with us until she was sure, but now she was convinced. *Something* had injured Graham's brain. She told us to be prepared for the possibility that Graham would never walk or ride a bike.

Soon we began to meet with the first of many kind people who work in various ways with children who are developing slowly. We learned that cerebral palsy can be mild or severe. At first we were certain that, if we worked hard with all those good people, Graham's disability would be mild. But Graham's CP was not mild. During the next twenty-two years, he would never feed himself or speak. He would never even roll over in bed without assistance.

"Don't know much about you
Don't know who you are
We were doing fine without you
But we could only go so far
Don't know why you chose us
Were you watching from above
Is there someone there who knows us
Said we'd give you all our love."
　　　　　　—Mark Cohn, "The Things We've Handed Down"

Cerebral palsy is a wastebasket term for a variety of conditions that injure nerves prior to or during birth. The injury can be mild or severe. Some individuals are affected so minimally that only the trace of a limp reveals damage to the brain or spinal cord. Other people, like Graham, have more profound damage to nerve cells and require wheelchairs and assistance with all of their daily activities. The cause of CP is frequently unknown. The human brain develops throughout a mother's pregnancy, unlike other organs that are nearly fully developed within the first ten weeks. Accordingly, a virus, a toxin or an unknown "insult" can damage the developing brain at any time during gestation, even when the mother feels healthy and is unaware of any illness.

Except for his frail legs, Graham looked physically perfect. His silky brown hair had auburn highlights that glistened in the sun. He had expressive hazel eyes, flawless skin that tanned beautifully and strong chest and shoulder muscles. His facial features and teeth were perfect. He never had a cavity or needed braces. But, like other children with severe

CP, Graham was nonverbal and it was difficult to be certain about his intellectual capacity. Some kids with cerebral palsy have mental retardation and others don't.

Until an individual learns a communication skill, it may be impossible to know exactly what his or her cognitive ability is. Those of us who have been around people with disabilities assume that the person is "all there" intellectually, even if he or she cannot communicate in a conventional way. In the heartening book and movie *My Left Foot,* Christy Brown reveals himself to be a remarkable artist and an intellect with an irreverent sense of humor, once his mother discovers that he is communicating quite profoundly with the movements of one foot.

Naturally, Cynthia and I wondered about Graham's mental capacity over the course of his life. Early on, according to the pediatrician's growth charts, his brain was discouragingly small, based on head circumference and, later, MRI scans that showed key brain areas were underdeveloped. But, even as we wondered about his cognitive status, we intuitively sensed that Graham could understand everything we said and treated him accordingly. His eyes were alert and sparkled with understanding, although it was not easy for him to focus steadily on us. There was something in his expressions that radiated both intelligence and kindness.

At some point, however, the term *mental retardation* began to appear in Graham's medical records and there was no highly scientific way to prove that the description was wrong. He had spasticity (tight muscles) and athetosis (writhing movements) that made it nearly impossible for him to control his body. It must have been profoundly frustrating for him when he attempted to use a computer switch that was activated by pushing a big red button—and his body simply would not cooperate. In one sense, Cynthia and I didn't care at all whether or not Graham was "retarded." We loved him unconditionally just the way he was and couldn't have loved him any more had he woken up one day, somersaulted out of bed, recited one of Hamlet's soliloquies and announced a cure for cancer.

The way we saw it, Graham was perfect, exactly as he was.

Until recently, I never gave much thought to how our brains process emotions. In Graham's case, I just knew that we loved to hug our son and that he loved to be hugged.

Not long ago, however, I stumbled upon the fascinating work of scientists at Johns Hopkins University called neurobiologists. The researchers were able to describe in detail the science behind our tactile sense, the tangible sensations that we receive from touching things in our environment. Nerves in the skin constantly convey information to the brain about what's happening on the surface of the body, including nuances of perception like pressure, motion, temperature and vibration. But, it turns out that humans also have a second, discrete sensory system for feeling and distinguishing *emotional touch*. That system even has its own nerve fibers called *C tactile fibers* and its own place in the brain where the signals are received, *the posterior insula*. So the distinct pleasure that humans feel during hugging and caressing apparently has a biological basis. The scientists have shown that emotional touch is crucial for normal development in babies, and many hospital neonatal units today have volunteer "huggers" for traumatized newborns.

It sounds as if the researchers are saying that love can quite literally be *felt*. And it is entirely possible that emotional touch remains necessary for psychological well-being throughout life. When Graham came along, Cynthia and I had never heard of C tactile fibers nor the posterior insula, but we instinctively used emotional touch just about every moment we were with our son. To stroke him and hug him came to us as naturally as breathing. Some of the time, we were able to interpret Graham's mood or energy level through physical contact. In the car, for example, Graham was rarely out of touch with the parent driving next to him. When he and I drove somewhere, my right hand and his left were communicating. Certain squeezes conveyed excitement and others meant, "Dad, I'm tired of being stuck in this damned seat! Get me the heck outta here!" At times Graham was also able to use his voice to express how he felt, using some lively vocalizations that did not quite form actual words.

When Cynthia and I pushed Graham in his stroller on walks, we were in constant touch with him, stroking his hair, rubbing his neck and positioning his legs. He, in turn, would subtly cradle one of our arms to indicate that he was enjoying himself or to let us know that it was time to head home.

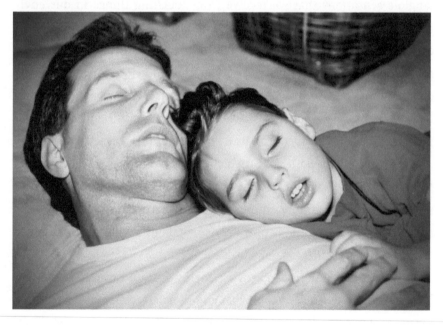

Emotional touch

I once asked a child psychologist who was a patient of mine how I would know if Graham was getting too old for all that touching.

"Don't worry about it," he said. "Graham will let you know if he's tired of it."

But, as Graham grew older, he never seemed to grow tired of it. He and I still took naps side-by-side and found comfort in one another's rhythmic breathing, curled up together like two spoons in a drawer. He always luxuriated in the vigorous hand and foot rubs that Cynthia gave him.

In time, Graham would become a camper at a magical summer camp for adults and children with disabilities on the island of Martha's Vineyard. Cynthia and I would ultimately spend time there, too, volunteering as cook and camp doctor. Camp Jabberwocky, as it is widely known, could easily serve as the definitive laboratory for the neurobiologists of Johns Hopkins, because emotional touch is everywhere there—and so is joy.

We told Graham many times a day how much he was adored and he heard and processed our words. But *touch*, perhaps more than anything else, defined the love that enveloped him.

Before we discovered Camp Jabberwocky, however, I had an opportunity to join the Massachusetts Special Olympics medical team for a couple of summers. That large, joyous group is passionately dedicated to Eunice Kennedy Shriver's idea of empowering people with disabilities through sports. Years later, Graham would become one of the millions of athletes around the world who participate in the friendly competitions that are dedicated to the inclusion of all people. When I decided to volunteer, Graham was still just two years old. Cynthia and I were becoming aware that he might be quite disabled and, for the first time, I wanted to explore the possibility of assisting people with disabilities in some capacity and to learn more about them. I noticed a flier in the hospital where I worked, indicating that the Massachusetts Special Olympics summer games were coming up soon in Boston. I called their office to see if they needed a medical volunteer.

By chance, the group had recently lost its medical director and, much to my surprise, I was offered that position. Proudly—and naively, as I would soon learn—I drove down that same night to Massachusetts Institute of Technology, where the group's planning sessions took place. I walked into MIT's sprawling campus center on the Charles River on a warm summer evening and met the volunteer medical staff, which was led by a spirited and dedicated group of EMTs. Besides the paramedics, there were nurses, doctors, physical therapists and all kinds of students around tables in a huge lecture hall. Many of them had been volunteers for years, and I felt sheepish assuming my role as medical director, having paid no dues at all. But, after some good-natured teasing, the team welcomed me warmly.

We needed to be prepared to care for some 5,000 people, including athletes with a vast range of disabilities, their coaches and their families, for two nights and two days at sites all around the city of Boston. The logistics were formidable. Athletes and coaches would be staying in dorms at Boston University, while the competition venues were primarily across the Charles River at MIT and Harvard. Many of the participants were medically fragile and taking multiple medications. I worried about getting prescription drugs to them in a timely way when the athletes were going to be scattered around a city known for its paralyzing traffic.

We set up a command post at BU on Friday morning. The core group of EMTs had been through this before and were experts at organizing communications and logistics using two-way radios. We had about eighty medical volunteers in all, many with years of experience at these huge events. I was humbled to learn that some routinely worked twenty-four-hour shifts and vehemently refused to accept public recognition of any kind for their efforts. But, despite our preparations, when the athletes actually arrived later that afternoon, we were nearly overwhelmed. Hundreds of people with disabilities needed medications, inhaler treatments, and injections in the first few hours alone. Finding them in the initial chaos was formidable. Our tumultuous command center vibrated with the teeming mayhem of a Manhattan subway station at rush hour. Only the experience and diligence of the EMTs allowed us to survive those early hours without any major catastrophes. Many of the same firefighters stayed up all night, making sure that the needs of every athlete were met.

In the bedlam of the command center that Friday night, as the athletes were beginning to settle down in their dorm rooms, problems confronted us in rapid succession: A girl from western Massachusetts had forgotten to pack her seizure medications. A youngster with Down Syndrome was lost. Someone was having a panic attack in the lobby. A non-verbal boy with a rare genetic disorder was moaning on a cot and, when asked to evaluate him, I struggled uncomfortably to determine whether the problem was emotional or an actual medical emergency.

And, just moments before the opening ceremonies were to begin, we learned that the wheelchair of a tiny African American girl named Kylie, from the hardscrabble city of Brockton, Massachusetts, had been badly damaged when a truck carrying equipment from her area was involved in an accident. Kylie had severe cerebral palsy, but her heart was set on competing in a short track event for athletes able to push themselves in manual chairs. Her race was to be held the next morning, and her coach had just told her that her special competition chair was too badly damaged to use. Realizing that she would be unable to participate, the delicate ten-year-old with frail, flaccid legs was devastated. Over the clamor of the command center we could hear her sobs in the hall outside.

At some point during those frantic moments at Boston University, a strikingly handsome young EMT named Michael walked into the command center and asked me if he could volunteer. He lived and worked in Boston's vibrant Italian neighborhood, the North End. It was a beautiful Friday evening, and I pictured his carefree friends at a watering hole on Hanover Street celebrating the coming of summer to Boston. But the poised, athletic young man, for reasons of his own, had a different agenda that night. Michael had overheard Kylie's dilemma, and offered to assist. He tackled the problem of the broken wheelchair with singular determination, aware that her event was going to be held in the morning, with or without her.

Kylie's racing chair had high-tech carbon fiber wheels, and one of them was, in fact, irreparably damaged. No amount of jerry-rigging by Michael could fix it. The only way to make the chair work would be to find a replacement wheel. The hospital supply stores had closed and would not open again until the next morning, too late for the youngster from Brockton.

Michael, however, had no intention of accepting defeat that easily and he explained the situation to a Boston police officer on duty at the Opening Ceremonies. Together they hatched a plan. Making unofficial use of a police computer at the officer's precinct house, they found the name and phone number of the owner of a medical supply store in the Harvard Medical Area. They called the surprised proprietor at home, enlisted his collaboration and picked him up with a police escort, arriving at his store with the broken wheelchair at about midnight.

At 9 the next morning, Kylie participated in her race. Mike was on the sidelines of the MIT track, cheering her on after sleeping for three hours. The merchant from the hospital supply store was rumored to have been there, too. Like every athlete who has ever participated in the Special Olympics, Kylie was celebrated as a winner that day.

Two nights later, profoundly exhausted, I headed home, thinking about the people I had met that weekend, both the athletes and those who assisted them. As I drove out of the city toward the North Shore, I was stunned by what I had just witnessed. Following a stream of red taillights in the growing dusk, I sensed that something in me had begun to change.

When Graham was three years old, Cynthia and I made the decision to move from Marblehead to Los Angeles, reasoning that Graham's therapy would be more productive for him in a climate where he could be outdoors every day. I stumbled on a great job at the University of Southern California and Cynthia discovered opportunities to work as a stylist in Hollywood. During the four years we lived in Southern California, there were always calamities taking place, although longtime residents of the region handled them with equanimity. To newcomers from New England, however, the frequent disasters, large and small, were literally unsettling.

There were riots around the USC campus in South Central LA where I worked after Rodney King was beaten by members of the LAPD. There were mudslides in Malibu that washed homes into the Pacific, and flash fires from the Santa Ana winds on hillsides not far from where we lived. The Northridge earthquake, measuring 6.7 on the Richter Scale, shattered everything on our walls at 4:31 one morning. And, just when we thought things couldn't get more bizarre, we watched the infamous "Slow Speed O.J. Simpson White Bronco Chase."

However, within the small clinic where I worked at USC, there was harmony. We were a diverse collection of about a hundred people. Our heritage seemed to be nearly equal parts European, African, Asian and Latin American, with a few individuals from exotic places like Cyprus thrown in. We simply got along. We worked together effectively and celebrated the "mosaic" that we formed, marking everyone's birthdays with brief, but raucous parties and supporting one another when adversity struck.

One of our clinic's administrators was Anita Hodge, an exuberant and irrepressible African American resident of South Central LA. What I knew of Watts was a caricature of racial tension and gang wars between the Bloods and Crips. Anita was the first person I had met who actually lived there. This dynamo of a woman was one of the first to welcome me when I arrived to serve as executive director of the clinic and, despite our very different backgrounds, we soon became friends. Anita met Graham and Cynthia and, after a month or two, I learned that my family was on the prayer list at her church.

Anita was part of a group she called the "prayer warriors," people who rallied spiritually for anyone facing adversity. In the beautiful phrase of Jay Austin, the champion of openheartedness who was killed with his girlfriend by ISIS while bicycling in Asia, Anita was a "merchant in the gift economy." Someone who demonstrates every day that people are inherently kind. One day, Anita's effervescent daughter, Kenita, age eleven, came by the clinic, knocked on my door and personally told me not to worry. She herself had placed Graham's name on the altar at their church.

Friends from the East would occasionally contact me and ask if I was worried at all about working in the middle of South Central LA, given its history of violence.

"No, not really. Not when we have friends here who have us in their prayers."

In the—mostly—friendly competition to determine which parent was the more colorful and prolific creator of nicknames for their only child, Graham's mother was the runaway winner. Led by her, we may have set a record for the number of goofy terms of endearment that two parents can come up with for one child. Very early on Graham was "Peeper" and "Baby Doll." For a long time I called him "Bud," but then it was "Buddy" and, later on, "Budafer," while, to his mom, he was "Laddie," or "Laddifer." When we were roughhousing, he was "Goon" or "Dirtball" until the two combined one day into "Goonball." Cynthia often addressed her son as "Best Little Man in the World," but that was shortened to "Manny," which then expanded to "Manny Man," before finally, and improbably, morphing into "Manaschevitz."

After seeing *The Motorcycle Diaries*, I called Graham "Fuser" (Few-say) or "Ernesto." On those occasions I thought of myself as "Alberto."

That said, I freely acknowledge that Graham's mom was the undisputed queen of whimsical sobriquets for our boy. After not seeing him for an extended time—two or even three minutes—his mom would greet her son as if she hadn't seen him in years with euphoric terms of endearment, strung together seamlessly in a single breath, as in:

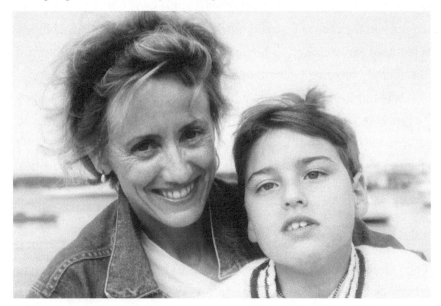

Cynthia with "Punkus Aurelius"

"Well! Hello, my best friend, the best person in the world, my sweet pea, my peapod, my handsome dude, my gorgeous man, the man of my dreams, my lovie, my loviest love, my sweet man, the sweetest man in the world!"

When he was a little older, Cynthia started calling Graham "Punk" or "Punkin' Pie," which then evolved into "Punkus Aurelius." To his adoring mother, our boy was part rock star, part pastry and part Roman Emperor.

Cynthia came up with the idea of enrolling Graham in a Challenger Little League near our home in Pasadena, a softball program for youngsters with special needs. He had great fun there. Cynthia's cherished friend of many years, the irrepressible, twinkling Johnny Everts, came down from Northern California to help Graham bat and field during one of his very first ball games. Johnny was Graham's on-field "buddy" or helper that day and they swung the bat together with unbridled energy. Johnny, who had not had the chance to spend much time around kids with disabilities, called it an "awakening," as he ran to first base, cheered on by jubilant fans, literally carrying Graham in his arms.

It was fun to see Graham in a baseball uniform. He seemed to enjoy the games in which many youngsters "run the bases" in wheelchairs and walkers, assisted by families, coaches and friends. At the Challenger Little League, kids were assigned randomly to teams with Major League names.

Graham was a member of the Angels.

When Graham was four or five years old, Cynthia took him for a walk in his jogger at a park in Los Angeles. As they stopped to have a drink and admire a striking flower, the Bird of Paradise, a stranger approached them. She was an older woman with a whimsical face, who looked like the actress Ruth Gordon when she played eccentric characters in the latter part of her career. Squatting down to Graham's level and looking at him keenly, she said, "This boy has the light of God in his eyes."

Cynthia told me about the incident later that day. Graham had a knack for attracting people in seemingly random situations like that. During the same period of time, I took a photo in our living room of Graham as he was held by Cynthia while he gazed upward. There was a warm, gossamer light shining on his face. Looking at the print later, I had a strange impression that the light was *coming* from Graham's face and shining outward. The photo would become one of our all-time favorite images of him.

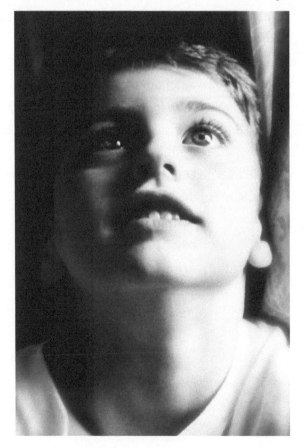

Several years later, I took a photo of Graham sleeping in the stern of a rowboat on the Concord River in Massachusetts. The glossy print that was made from it had a curious optical effect that once again gave me pause. I assumed it was some kind of chemical artifact from the printing process, but it looked as if there was a huge arc of light above the boat, a kind of halo. I noticed unusual lighting effects in other photos of our young hero over the years and generally attributed them to optical curiosities. One was a photo taken of the two of us skiing together in New England, with a brilliant sunburst seemingly shining directly down upon us. Another was the photo we used on the memory card at Graham's memorial service. It shows him gazing out of the passenger window of my car, greeting our lovely friend from Nigeria, Jane Unaeze, then a Harvard medical student. The light on his face seems ethereal, even celestial.

Cynthia and I are not people who find images of the Virgin Mary in our coffee grounds—no offense to those who do—so we are open to the idea that there may be scientific explanations for the visual phenomena in the photographs. But, even if there are plausible optical reasons for those effects, it does not change the conviction that Cynthia and I share with so many people who met our boy, including the stranger in the park in Los Angeles: Graham had the light of God in his eyes.

2

DRIVERS AND DUCKLINGS

*"My whole class in the fourth grade knew that Graham
could understand. And they were all his friends."*
                    —Charlotte Twaalfhoven

After four years in Southern California, Cynthia and I made the painful decision to end our marriage and return to New England. We would continue, however, to work together as Graham's advocates and true believers. After returning from LA, Graham shared time between his mother's home in Marblehead and my home in nearby Salem. At the age of eight, Graham became a pioneer in "inclusion" at the Bell School in Marblehead, thanks to the constant advocacy of his mom and the enthusiastic support of Special Education Director Bob Belucci, Principal Bob Farrell and his home room teachers, Joanne Mahalski and Maddie Cormier. Graham was, by far, the most disabled child the school had ever attempted to include in a traditional classroom setting. Special education is a hot-button topic in the school systems of small towns, and it required strong and thoughtful leadership within the Marblehead school system to make Graham's inclusion succeed.

Happily, the children at the Bell School accepted Graham unconditionally and treated his presence in their midst as something natural. A
few in particular—Katharine, Margaret, Alex, Charlotte ("Lotte"), Daria,
Matt and Teddy—intuitively sensed his intelligence and benevolence,
even at that young age. Those youngsters would become Graham's inner
circle and lifelong advocates. Like his parents, they knew that Graham's
brain was able to process everything going on around him, even though
he could not speak or control his body consistently. Despite the support
of his attentive young friends, however, introducing a boy with serious
disabilities into the daily routine of a middle school *was* challenging.
Accommodating a youngster who was nonverbal and had significant
medical issues, including epilepsy, raised some concerns. It was Maddie,
his homeroom teacher, who came up with a creative concept as Graham
began fourth grade that proved to be a perfect ice breaker and paved the
way for integrating Graham into the mainstream of middle school culture. She christened it the *Designated Driver.*

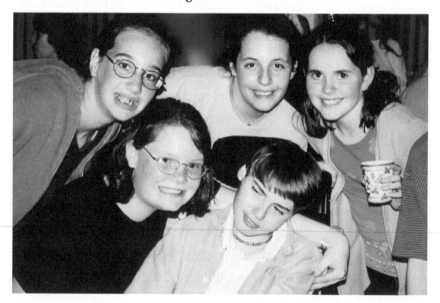

Graham with some of his "drivers."

Each day this serene woman named three students in Graham's home-room to be his designated drivers for the day. Their job was to share the responsibility of pushing him in his wheelchair to all activities, including assemblies and recess, while interacting closely with Graham's exuberant one-to-one aide, Beth Crowe. Although Maddie's belief in the concept lessened any angst that existed among the school staff, a few concerns persisted: What if the kids resented this new responsibility? Would it embarrass Graham to have cute girls his age pushing him around? Were the kids simply too young to understand the satisfaction that comes with assisting another person?

Very quickly it became clear that those concerns were inconsequential. The Designated Driver concept was an unqualified success! Far from being an awkward job for a youngster of nine or ten, pushing Graham became a coveted role, thanks to his magnetism and the compassionate example set by his popular "drivers."

On Graham's tenth birthday, we arranged for his whole class to go out on the Charles River in Boston on a "Duck Tour" in one of the silly-looking amphibious boats that kids and tourists love. Maddie asked every student in her class to try to clear their calendars on that weekend day in order to celebrate as a group with Graham. Only one classmate could not attend. Cassidy Goodwin had a karate competition that she had prepared for enthusiastically, and it could not be rescheduled. On the Friday before the Duck Tour, the pretty youngster with silky brown hair and hazel eyes walked over to Graham and told him she would win the tournament—for him.

Despite chilly weather, the Duck Tour was "awesome," according to Graham's young guests. Even the boat's captain went out of his way to make sure Graham was enjoying the day, allowing him to steer the vessel for a while, with assistance. Cynthia and I sat back and marveled at the most exquisite gift that Graham received that day: the genuine friendship of his peers. The following Monday, during a break between classes,

Cassidy Goodwin stood up among her classmates. Pulling a huge trophy from her backpack, she walked over to Graham, smiled broadly and said, "This is for you, my friend. Happy Birthday!

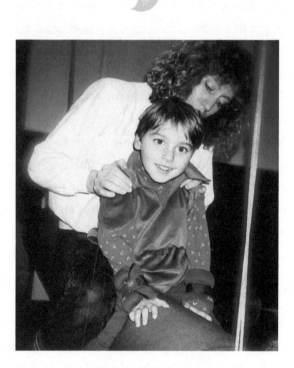

Graham with Eileen

On weekends, we took Graham for physical therapy at an inspired little clinic in a drab mini-mall near the big reservoir in Woburn, Massachusetts. His therapist there, Eileen Ladwig, had a knack for getting Graham to give his best, and he made great strides with her, improving his motor tone, posture and flexibility. It was marvelous to watch them work together on mats and a big swinging canvas log that Eileen had improvised. To get to the clinic required driving on Interstate 95, known as Route 128 in Massachusetts, one of the most congested and unmerciful stretches of highway in all of America. Fortunately, most of our trips to Woburn were on weekends, when traffic was slightly less pernicious.

On one memorable Monday morning at rush hour, I found myself crawling along Route 128, late for a meeting at a convention center outside Boston. I was alone in my Jeep Grand Cherokee, but in the immediate company of what felt like thousands of other frustrated motorists. Subliminally, I became aware that I was passing the reservoir in Woburn where I had watched Graham doing his PT two days earlier, and I pictured him concentrating and trying his best to follow Eileen's instructions. The image filled me with pride. Smiling from that memory, I became aware that the traffic was slowing even more, if that was even possible. I was in the high-speed lane—at that moment an oxymoron—and the line of vehicles in front of me was maneuvering around something adjacent to the Jersey barrier that formed the median of the massive roadway.

A moment later, the cause of the slowdown came into view: a mother mallard duck and a dozen fuzzy yellow ducklings were anxiously waddling south, single file. They were trapped between the cement barrier and the unrelenting line of cars and trucks moving at a crawl just inches from their rapidly shuffling, bright orange webbed feet. Nobody was stopping. Cars and thundering tractor trailers, air brakes rasping, were squeezing by the ducks and resuming their place in the bumper to bumper, gas-guzzling procession that stretched far to the south.

Until I stopped. With no conscious thought process, I drove about ten yards ahead of the mother duck, got out and managed to simultaneously stop her and the five lanes of rush hour traffic beside me. It took a few moments to convince the frightened bird to allow me to escort her brood across the highway, under the guard rail along Route 128, and into the safety of the marsh next to the road. As they disappeared into that wetland, I experienced a very weird feeling that somehow this mother duck knew that deliverance for her family had arrived when I got out of my car.

Walking back across the asphalt, I had the fleeting feeling that my mind and body had come loose. My Jeep suddenly looked very peculiar, parked in the high-speed lane of an interstate highway. Five lanes of snarled traffic had backed up about a quarter of a mile.

Shockingly, not a single car or truck had moved. Those merciless commuters—some of whom would cheerfully strangle Mother Teresa (if she were still alive) rather than allow a single car to squeeze in front of them—were waiting for me to reach my vehicle before proceeding. In my out-of-body state, I resisted an impulse to do the squatting *duckwalk* across the road, the famous element of guitar showmanship created by Chuck Berry and adopted today by the country singer Keith Urban, among others. In the duckwalk, a musician stalks across the stage in a low stance, sometimes even hopping on one leg. But the urge passed, and I half-stumbled to the Jeep, fully expecting to be pancaked by a Winnebago.

But, as I hustled to my car, I noticed smiles on a few faces and even an appreciative wave or two. Moments later, a fanfare of friendly toots from horns ordinarily honked with animosity heralded my reentry to the highway as the other drivers allowed me to ease back into my lane and lead them off to the south.

At the meeting, I allowed myself to relive those moments on the highway with amusement and some pride. I wondered why I had stopped. I had given it no particular thought; I had just done it. Was it coincidental that the incident unfolded directly beside Graham's PT clinic? Or had I channeled my son subliminally? When the mallard and her family came into view, I had been thinking of his spunk and courage. Graham had a decency, even a nobility that was inspirational to those who knew him. His schoolmates frequently said that watching Graham made them want to try harder, to *be* better. Maybe that explains why I was the one who stopped that morning. Maybe there is no such thing as happenstance.

In retrospect, though, I should have done the duckwalk.

3

JABBERWOCKY

Jabberwocky...the Poem

"And hast thou slain the Jabberwock?
Come to my arms my beamish boy!
O frabjous day! Callooh Callay!
He chortled in his joy."

—Lewis Carroll, *Through the Looking Glass*

Jabberwocky...the Camp

"On an island off the southern coast of Massachusetts, there is a place where hope flourishes. The island is Martha's Vineyard. The place is Camp Jabberwocky, a small summer camp for the disabled situated in the woods not too far from Lake Tashmoo. Jabberwocky emerged in the early 1950s. It began in a time when public sentiment regarding the role of disabled people in society was dismal. Services were minimal and rights were not yet an issue. Nonetheless, Jabberwocky sprang forth. The camp started as a small experiment: a handful of children, a tiny summer cottage, a director and a young assistant. From there camp has grown to a fourteen-acre site, seventeen buildings and a large volunteer

staff. It now serves about one hundred children and adults every summer.

But this is only the beginning ..."

—*A Brief History of the Martha's Vineyard*
Cerebral Palsy Camp

I watched in awe as Pete Halby picked Graham up out of his wheelchair and threw him high into the golden afternoon sunlight that sparkled on dozens of triangular sails, far out on the cobalt blue waters of Nantucket Sound.

It was the first summer that my nine-year-old son and I were spending together at Camp Jabberwocky, and I was just beginning to realize that we had joined a kind of parallel universe, one that existed just six miles across the ocean from the world we left behind when we boarded the big ferry in Woods Hole earlier that same day. When we arrived on Martha's Vineyard that dazzling summer afternoon, Graham as a camper and I as a first-time camp physician, I had immediately noticed a hand-painted phrase on the back door of one of the camp minivans that greeted us at the dock in Vineyard Haven: "The best way to explain it is to do it." I remember wondering about that expression at the time and, while I have been a volunteer doctor at Camp Jabberwocky for many years now, I think I am just beginning to understand what it means.

Camp Jabberwocky is not easy to describe. It's a place where people with different abilities and disabilities come together for several weeks in a picture-postcard setting to share the fun of summer, test limits and experience life vividly. During their time on the island, the campers and counselors live in the present. Playfulness and whimsicality are celebrated. Outrageousness is encouraged. People who are seriously disabled are viewed as uniquely intriguing. By summer's end, compassion, laughter and love have turned an eclectic collection of individuals into a rambunctious extended family.

I knew little of Camp Jabberwocky that first day of the thirteen summer sessions I would ultimately spend there with my son. After arriving "on island," our loud camp entourage had boarded Camp's signature red bus and assorted minivans and headed straight to the beach for a cookout. The magnificent late June afternoon proclaimed summer's long-awaited arrival. At State Beach, the stunning sandy expanse on the northeast side of the island facing Nantucket Sound, the percussionist Rick Bausman and his spirited drum ensemble were set up in the sand playing Haitian and African-based rhythms. The sun was descending in the glowing sky behind us, giving a golden hue to the clear afternoon light. The air was warm and pungent as the smell of the sea mingled with the first barbecue scents of the season.

Campers were pushed and carried down to the beach, where dancing erupted instantly. Campers who could stand did so and pranced wildly with their counselors. Others danced with abandon while seated in their wheelchairs. Everyone was ready to boogie. It was my first lesson that letting go of inhibition is an integral part of the Jabberwocky experience. Pete Halby, an exuberant counselor and nonstop instigator of fun and mischief, had spent summers on the island throughout his life. I watched as he asked Graham if he wanted to join the dance. Although Graham was nonverbal, his eyes showed that he was up for it. My own eyes widened as Pete unbuckled Graham, picked him up out of his wheelchair and threw him in the air! Thus began an hour or so of improvisational dancing with Pete carrying Graham in his arms and intermittently tossing him up and catching him while they bopped around the circle of drummers, weaving among dozens of other revelers, each moving spontaneously in his or her unique fashion.

Wendy Grey, then a medical student, was carrying Scott Scherer, a youngster with cerebral palsy, who was beaming from ear to ear, and I watched with fascination as the pair danced merrily at the edge of the gentle surf. In that golden hour before sunset, everyone seemed to be cavorting without the slightest self-consciousness.

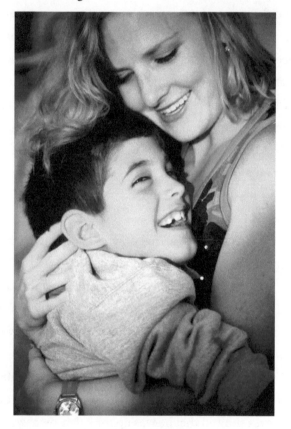

Wendy and Scott

I looked over at Graham, bouncing crazily in Pete's arms. He looked back at me with a giant grin on his face, as if to say, "Dad ... the best way to explain it is to do it!"

One warm early summer evening just after sunset, I was feeling slightly grumpy. I had been at the camp all day, and I was tired from the frenetic activity and the intense emotions that I always feel there. While those feelings are powerfully positive, they can be draining sometimes. Just as I was about to go back to what was then referred to as the "Doctor's House," a small home that Camp Jabberwocky owns just down the street, ready to slump on the couch and watch the end of a Red Sox game, one of the counselors asked me to check on a camper in Bandersnatch. (The cabins are named after characters from the famous Lewis Carroll poem about the Jabberwock.) She was concerned about an impish youngster named Jonah. He had CP and depended on others for all his daily needs.

Jonah had severe spasticity and was in the habit of sleeping on his belly, insisting with grimaces that it was the only way that he could be comfortable in bed. As a result, though, he had developed painful sores on the front of his lower thighs and kneecaps. I trudged up to see him in the twilight of that perfect June evening. Cicadas were buzzing. There was a gentle breeze in the scrub oaks that shelter the campus. I could faintly hear the lyrical pinging of a bell buoy out in Vineyard Haven harbor. Lights were on in the cabins around Camp, and I could hear muted chatter, laughter and some singing from cabins in the distance.

After seeing Jonah's abrasions, I decided to apply antibiotic ointment to the scraped areas, dress them with a nonstick bandage and repeat that procedure for the next few nights. I went back out to gather the supplies from our modest clinic in the main cabin. As I walked, I wondered what I was doing. It was a glorious summer evening on one of the most beautiful islands in the world. I imagined that, at that very moment, some of my old school pals might be sitting on the deck of a big, beautiful boat in Edgartown Harbor, sipping gin and tonics and looking up at the stars with not a care in the world. I envisioned well-heeled vacationers laughing by candlelight over lobster dinners in elegant night spots around the island.

By contrast, I was dirty and exhausted, about to visit a hot cabin on a trivial first-aid mission for a disabled kid from Indiana whom I had never even heard speak. And, like almost everyone at camp, I was a volunteer. If I was going to take care of people during my precious vacation time, wouldn't it be smarter to do something that involved getting paid? In that grouchy state of mind, I opened the creaky screen door to Bandersnatch and sat on the edge of Jonah's wooden bunk. A faint scent of Coppertone and wet towels hung in the still air of the cabin. In the semidarkness, it didn't take long to apply the ointment and dressings and turn the youngster back on his belly. I said a cursory "Good night" and pushed open the screen door to leave. But just as the door closed, I thought I heard a sound coming from Jonah's bunk.

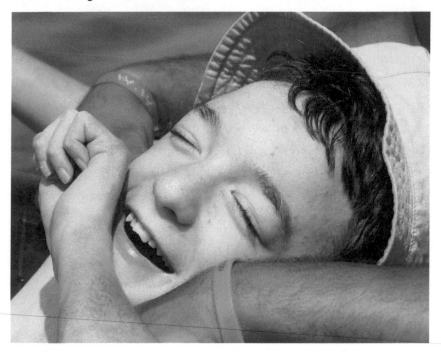

Jonah

I went back in.

"Jonah, did you say something?"

Indeed, in a faint, halting voice delivered with great effort, I heard him speak for the first time.

"Ankyoo Dahdhastee."

"What's that, Jonah? I didn't quite hear you."

"Ankyoo Dahdastee."

"Jonah, I'm sorry. I'm not understanding you. Try one more time."

On his third try, I finally got it. In one of my life's most wondrous epiphanies, I clearly heard Jonah say:

"Thank you, Doctor Steve."

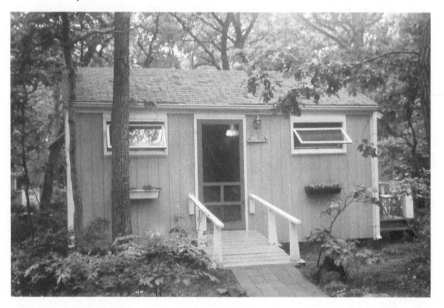

Jonah's Cabin

In the poignant moments that followed, I felt the full pathos of Jonah's condition. There was no denying that his circumstances were challenging. But we were together at Camp Jabberwocky, where it is difficult to be gloomy for long. I sat for a few moments marveling at the grace of the little boy lying patiently on his belly in the twilight and rubbed the back of his head.

"You're very welcome, Jonah. We'll do the same thing tomorrow night. I hope you have a good sleep."

As I pushed open the screen door of Bandersnatch for the final time that evening and emerged into that splendid summer night, I was not jealous of anyone in the world. I knew that I was exactly where I was meant to be.

"Jabberwocky is a community. It has families and extended families and grandparents and children. It has births and deaths and marriages. It has oral history, traditions, myths, and legends. It has people with a full range of abilities, skills, and interests. And these people work, play, eat, and create together. They argue and dance together. They write and cry together. And, like people in other communities, they are here year after year. A few come and go each season, but the majority are here living together every summer."
—A Brief History of the Martha's Vineyard
Cerebral Palsy Camp

Graham had been a Jabberwocky camper for several summers when an old friend of mine and his family came to the Vineyard for a vacation and stopped to see us at Camp. An unwritten rule there is that everyone is welcome to visit, as long as they get up in front of the entire camp and tell a story, preferably an embarrassing and salty one about themselves. Afterward, typically amid wild cheering, they are heartily welcomed into Camp's increasingly vast extended family. While my friend, Charlie, was waiting to address everyone at dinner, I looked around at the mayhem in the main cabin that serves as our dining room. I marveled, as I often do, at what I saw all around me in that unremarkable space. An abundance of uninhibited affection was on display at every table. And so was an irreverent spirit of shared silliness that has characterized Camp since its inception in 1953.

As always, the room was overflowing with the exuberance of people who simply accept one another and know that they belong together, that exquisite feeling called the "opposite of loneliness" by the late Marina Keegan. And, not least of all, among the giggling groups at every table, and even in the raucous dishwasher room, I could simply *feel* the uniquely tender connection among us all that has come to be called "Jabberwocky Love."

When his turn came, my old schoolmate told a funny anecdote about a misadventure we had experienced on a road trip across the country in a borrowed car. It was a good story met with enthusiastic laughter and applause. He and I got together later and talked about the improbable twists and turns our lives had taken since those days of yesteryear. In a kind way, he said, "Steven, this place is really wonderful. I'm glad that you and Graham are part of it. Thank God it's here for kids like these. It's just too bad, because of their disabilities, that they can't go to a regular camp and do all the stuff that able-bodied kids get to do."

I thought about his comment for a moment, knowing that he meant it in a kind way. But Charlie was clearly missing a few things. First of all, with the boisterous assistance of their counselors, the Jabberwocky campers find ways to do just about everything that "able-bodied" kids do—and then some. More importantly, my friend had not yet fully appreciated the magical celebration that was going on in that noisy cabin in the woods on the outskirts of Vineyard Haven.

"Charlie, you may be right. But it's even more unfortunate that all the able-bodied kids in the world can't come to Camp Jabberwocky."

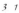

It was an overcast day right after the Fourth of July, about two weeks after camp started. One of the campers, Cathy DiSciullo, was sitting in a beach chair on the far edge of our big group at State Beach and fell over. It was not a violent fall, just a slow motion flop to the side. It was not the sort of thing that would hurt her, but, with Cathy's limited use of her arms and legs due to an autoimmune disorder, she would be stuck on her side in the sand for a while until assistance arrived. I happened to be standing in the back of the group, near the cookout grills, and I had a clear view of the scene. After Cathy fell over, or, more accurately, it seemed to me, *as* she was falling over, I watched four or five counselors react and reflexively move in her direction. What struck me about their reaction was that about half of the responders did not appear to have had even a peripheral view of Cathy from where they were sitting or lying in the sand. Yet, they had appeared to react just as instantaneously as the counselors with a direct view of her falling.

I saw this unfold right in front of me, and I can't explain it scientifically. It was like watching a flock of birds banking, en masse, in the same split second, or a school of fish, composed of a thousand individual creatures, instantly changing direction in unison. Perhaps it should not have surprised me. Each Camp Jabberwocky group develops an almost mystical bond during the long summer days spent together. After a while, the counselors seem to *sense* whatever needs to be done, and they simply do it without apparent thought. As the sign painted on that Camp van says, "The best way to explain it is to do it."

Scientists have tried to figure out the communication of the birds, the fish and even colonies of ants, but they are not at all sure how it works. Thought transference? Electromagnetic signaling? Nobody knows. (If you think about it, how *would* a scientist know what a carpenter ant is thinking?) But in those species, it seems that certain actions are no longer the property of a single individual, but of a group as a whole. Individuals flourish, and even survive, precisely because they are part of a larger *community.* As I pondered that mysterious connection among the birds and fish, I noticed a group of sandpipers darting in and out of the gentle surf in unison, right in front of Cathy Disciullo's favorite spot on the beach.

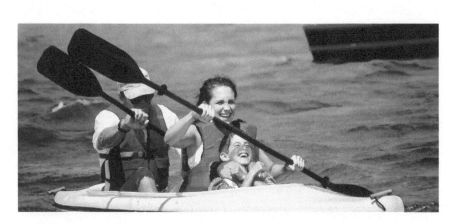

Sengekontacket

In our early years at Camp, the Jabberwocky family met an inspired and fun-loving group called AccesSportAmerica. That spirited bunch of athletes would reveal to Graham and me the possibility of participating in high-challenge sports together. AccesSportAmerica was founded in 1995 by the Reverend Ross Lilley, supported by his wife Jean, his daughter Hanna, and his son Josh, who had been born with cerebral palsy in 1984 and could not walk on his own. The Lilleys' pioneering idea was to create a water sports program that would be available to anyone with a disability. Since his son's infancy, Ross had invented ways for Josh to get out on the water with him. Windsurfing had long been a passionate hobby for Ross, and he wanted to share it with his son. The adapted windsurfer he created, featuring a chair for Josh, was the catalyst for equipment innovations they would create later in sports like cycling and skiing. Finding a way for Josh to enjoy windsurfing changed the course of the Lilleys' lives and, ultimately, the lives of scores of people—with and without disabilities.

In 1996, early in its existence, AccesSportAmerica brought high-challenge water sports to Camp Jabberwocky for the first time. The setting was a sparkling three-mile-long body of shallow water on the north-east side of the island, just inside the barrier beach that faces Nantucket Sound. Close to the road, free of big waves and dotted with sand bars and salt marshes, the coastal lagoon was the perfect setting to introduce exhilarating water sports to the campers of Jabberwocky. Sengekontacket is the lyrical name the Native Americans gave to that place of transcendent beauty. For a few days, hoping to make even a small contribution to this new Jabberwocky adventure, I minimally helped the AccesSport team on the water and on the beach. I was by no means an accomplished windsurfer, but I was experienced enough to stay out of the water—most of the time. Along with the Jabberwocky counselors, I helped load campers on and off windsurfers, kayaks and inner tubes.

Then, on a magnificent day in early July, with a light onshore breeze, Ross asked if I wanted to take Graham out on the special windsurfer with the seat attached to its board that he had invented for Josh. My heart soared! We strapped Graham into the seat, donned life vests and pushed off into Sengekontacket under the watchful eyes of Ross and his team. The wind was light and the special board was stable. The water sparkled around us. As I stood, straddling Graham's chair, arms wrapped around him, we tacked toward Edgartown for a while and then came about and rode the downwind leg back toward Farm Neck, on the Oak Bluffs side of the pond. As we glided through the calm water that morning, Graham was able to briefly place his hands over mine on the "boom" and experience the feeling of controlling our sail.

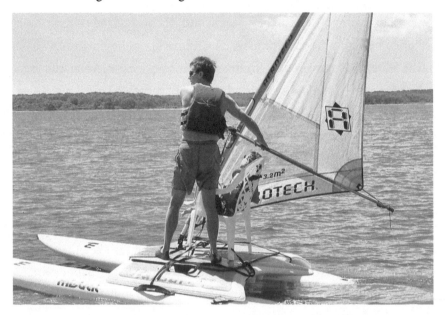

My son and I shared something sublime in those moments. The exquisite beauty of the setting, the warmth of the sun and the thrill of moving together over the water, powered only by the wind, combined to make it an indelible, transformative experience. On the lagoon that morning Graham and I discovered a new and breathtaking sense of freedom. We were proud to have participated in a challenging sport and we sensed that we had moved in harmony with a stunning sliver of the natural world. For both of us, it would be the most thrilling athletic experience of a lifetime. Thanks to that early inspiration from AccesSportAmerica, Graham and I later learned to ski, kayak and cycle together on modified equipment. Each of those sports was wonderful for us in its own way. But nothing would ever compare to that morning on Sengekontacket when we rode the wind together on Ross and Josh's windsurfer.

Later that summer, Graham and I went with the rest of the campers to a secluded beach in the scenic village of Chilmark, on the northwest coast of the Vineyard, to meet up with Ross and his AccesSportAmerica team. It was a warm, cloudless summer day. The Elizabeth Islands, just a few miles to the west across Vineyard Sound, were shimmering on the horizon. Ross and his gang arrived directly from Cape Cod, crossing the six miles of Vineyard Sound in a pair of water-ski boats. They brought along a set of skis that Ross had adapted for Josh, along with specially designed windsurfers, kayaks and a huge inner tube.

The pair of skis that Ross had rigged for his son had bindings for *two* athletes. The front set of bindings had been designed for Josh, then about eleven years of age, who could only stand with support. Our Jabberwocky gang shared a moment of anticipation as the father and son prepared to give us a demonstration. The boisterous camp group watched from the beach as Josh was helped into the bindings in knee-high water and leaned back into his father's muscular body. With his own feet in the back pair of bindings, Ross wrapped his arms around Josh and grabbed the handle of the ski rope, balancing their bodies in the choppy water and waiting for the moment of equilibrium when he would signal to the driver of the boat to hit the throttle. Suddenly, implausibly, Ross and Josh rose up out of the water and exploded off into the sound. The boat's powerful motor screamed ahead of them while plumes of spray from their single set of skis formed sparkling arcs against the morning sky. After a collective gasp of astonishment from our group on the shore, raucous cheering erupted, loud even by the tempestuous standards of Camp Jabberwocky.

It required amazing strength and freakish balance for Ross and Josh to pull off this remarkable athletic feat. It also took inspiration, imagination and, not least of all, the love and trust that bound a father and son. After demonstrating this astonishing water-skiing technique with Josh, Ross took out a number of other campers who were physically able to handle that level of exertion. The rest of his crew helped Graham and the others to kayak, windsurf or just enjoy floating on an inner tube in the shallow water on that protected corner of the island.

I had hopped up on the stern of the ski boat to get some photos and I had a perfect view of all the action. To my amazement, I was watching people who couldn't walk—or even stand by themselves—water-skiing on Vineyard Sound! Leaning into Ross, they were roaring along behind us, carving "rooster tails" of saltwater and foam, their wet skin sparkling with golden flecks of sunlight reflected off the churning water. Each time the boat slowed to drop a skier back at the beach, I saw wide grins and heard spontaneous, proud shouts. I recognized those shouts as the exuberant expressions of athletes who have just achieved a "personal best." For the campers who skied with Ross, it was an athletic experience that, quite likely, they had never even dreamed was possible.

Watching that scene and shaking my head, I was reminded of a remark attributed to the legendary Texas golf pro, Harvey Penick: "If you couldn't get a thrill out of that, you're pretty hard to get a thrill out of ..."

"The only thing that really changes the world is when somebody gets the idea that love can abound and can be shared."
—Reverend Fred Rogers,
Mister Rogers' Neighborhood

Several years ago, the Boston Celtics gave their "Heroes Among Us" award to Helen Lamb, Camp Jabberwocky's irrepressible founder, then in her early nineties. Helen's unique life ended at the age of ninety-seven when she died of natural causes at her home on the Vineyard. Her stated goal had been to die on her birthday and, consistent with her singular willfulness to do things her own way, she passed away on the anniversary of her birth in England.

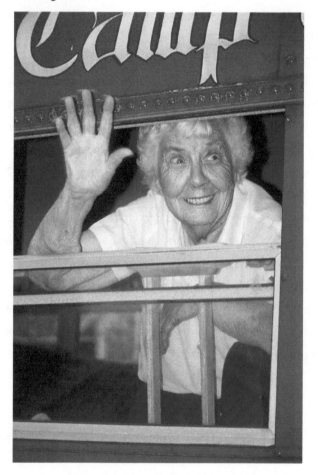

Helen Lamb

"Heroes Among Us" is a community outreach program that honors "individuals who have made an overwhelming impact on the lives of others." Helen had surely done that, creating both Camp Jabberwocky itself and a philosophy that has influenced nearly everyone who has visited her iconic creation in the woods of Vineyard Haven. Her idea was to give people with disabilities the chance to experience the joys of summer at the seashore, while challenging them to create a community in which they dare to try new experiences and laugh at themselves. Helen was a force of nature with no patience for social convention. She happily disregarded conventional wisdom entirely when it got in the way of her vision for what she simply referred to as "Jabberwocky."

A widow with three small children when she arrived from England, Helen settled in the factory town of Fall River, Massachusetts. She worked as a speech therapist, driving daily to the homes of children with communication difficulties. As she watched young clients with cerebral palsy spending summers indoors, sitting in the dim parlors of their parents' homes, something changed in Helen. The realization that these kids rarely saw the light of day did more than bother her—it made her angry. She decided to find a location where, like any other children, youngsters with disabilities could experience the delights of summertime in New England. She had a premonition that an island not far off the coast of Massachusetts was destined to be that place.

Helen wanted her clients with cerebral palsy—initially including Larry Perry, Manny Furtado and Paul Remy—to feel the sun on their skin, to experience the invigorating shock of being dunked in the cold saltwater of the ocean and to savor every scent and flavor of a summer cookout. Nobody was going to stop her. And nobody did. On a wing and a prayer, she took several children with disabilities to a small cottage called "Happy Days" on Martha's Vineyard in the summer of 1953. She had a young assistant, little money and only a vague idea of what might happen after the ferry deposited her unusual group on the dock at Oak Bluffs. She had an instinct, though, that the people of the island would support her idea and would lend a hand when assistance was needed. That faith was quickly confirmed, as she explained in this note written in the early days of that first summer:

"Here we are with almost all we could wish for. The greatest relief for me is that we have plenty of food. The swings, see-saws and plenty of room are all here. As one of the older children said, 'We have only to wish for something and, in the morning it is here.'"

Helen's determination and, perhaps more so, her aggressive driving habits, earned her the nickname "Hellcat." Her irreverent sense of humor became legendary on the island and can be appreciated in her remarks published by the *Martha's Vineyard Times* following an award ceremony held on the island in 2009:

> "Before I left for the states, I spent time right after World War II in London digging up bodies from the rubble left by all the bombing. I closed their eyes and went on to the next until I found someone alive. One day we found a little girl alive who, for the longest time, would not talk to anyone. She just sat in a big chair. Then one day, probably feeling a bit frustrated, I lifted her up and said, 'For God's sake, Mary, say something.'
>
> She looked at me and said, 'Put me down!!!'"

Jabberwocky has a tradition of "winter follies," occasional gatherings during the dreary winter months that reunite campers and volunteers and keep the Camp spirit alive. Watching the Boston Celtics on TV on a particularly bleak January day, Graham and I came up with the idea for a new winter folly—a gathering of campers and volunteers at an NBA basketball game. Camp Jabberwocky has had a close relationship with the Boston Celtics over the years, based on its friendship with managing partner Wyc Grousbeck (the father of Graham's counselor, Kelsey). When we presented our idea to Wyc and the Celtics, they quickly embraced it.

Jabberwocky has been treated royally by the team ever since, on what has become an annual midwinter outing at the Boston Garden.

The Heroes Among Us award is presented several times per season during a television time-out in the second half of a game. Wyc arranged it so that Camp's winter folly would coincide with Hellcat's honor. By tradition, the recipient of the award is escorted onto the famed parquet floor of the Boston Garden and greeted by the captain of the Celtics. The PA announcer then briefly describes the achievements of the honoree. The entire ceremony takes place during the space of a single TV commercial break. Well—Hellcat hadn't quite understood that!

She had, in fact, prepared a theatrical five-minute acceptance speech, anticipating an opportunity to tell a live audience of 17,000 fans all about the history of Camp Jabberwocky. Helen expected that the game would be suspended during her address and launched into her speech with the impeccable diction of a veteran of the English stage. As the TV time-out wound down, it fell to a frantic Celtics public relations executive to gently pull her off the court and disabuse her of the idea that she would be addressing the big crowd at greater length. Our large Camp contingent watched the ceremony from the loftiest balcony in the building, affectionately known as "the Halo." That special open-seating area is perfect for fans in wheelchairs, but so high above the court that the giant players below look like Lilliputian versions of themselves. Fortunately, a massive Jumbotron hangs over the court and its enormous high-definition screen made it possible for us to clearly see and hear the award presentation. In addition, a hand-held camera up in the Halo section periodically captured animated Camp faces engaged in a variety of antics and projected them on the Jumbotron, much to our delight.

Hellcat had many strong personal beliefs that some people today might consider old-fashioned: One should look the other person in the eye during conversation! One should grip the hand of the other person firmly during a handshake! One should speak crisply and confidently! She had formed these convictions early on, during her years as a young actress in London, and she demanded that all individuals associated with Camp adhere to them or suffer her wrath. During the ceremony, when she shook the hand of the Celtics captain, Paul Pierce, who had by then earned roughly $180 million in a Hall of Fame career, we watched the Jumbotron and listened as Hellcat said:

"Son, that's a weak handshake. You'll never make anything of yourself with a grip like a dead fish!"

Like any upscale vacation destination, there are several spectacular golf courses on Martha's Vineyard. Near Camp, in a quiet enclave known as West Chop, sits Mink Meadows, a woodsy nine-hole layout in a secluded corner of the island overlooking Vineyard Sound. I befriended the golf pro there one year and hatched an idea to bring a few campers over to the course some evening at dusk. The plan was to select four or five campers who could walk and behave themselves reasonably well and have a quiet outing on the putting green. I was proud that I had thought of a new camp activity, even though it would benefit only a handful of the more able-bodied campers. Gillian Butchman, Hellcat's daughter, was camp director that year, and, as it turned out, she and I miscommunicated rather spectacularly about my plan for the outing at Mink Meadows.

On the appointed evening, I waited at the club for a single van to arrive with a handful of aspiring, well-mannered golfers who would engage in a gentlemanly—and ladylike—putting contest. My jaw dropped when I saw the entire camp arriving en masse in the big red bus, trailed by multiple minivans carrying, in total, some seventy-five or so wildly boisterous individuals.

A foursome was finishing its round on the last hole when the cacophonous assemblage approached from the parking lot in an invasion of walkers and wheelchairs. While a few ambulatory campers ran about wildly, the whole Camp entourage converged on the green. Needless to say, our group was blissfully ignorant of golf etiquette, or, more accurately, etiquette in general. As I watched in shock, it looked like a kind of assault was taking place on the previously discreet haven of Mink Meadows. The foursome was good-natured about the surprise ending to its round, and Camp proceeded to congregate around the practice green. We were able to borrow enough putters and balls from the greenskeeper to allow for a highly spirited putting contest among the cabins.

At one point, a tiny camper with cerebral palsy named Madison, standing only with the strong support of her counselor, stroked a curling twenty-foot putt directly into the heart of a cup. The Camp gathering exploded in a roar that was probably heard across Vineyard Sound on the coast of Rhode Island. Jabbwerwocky's putting contest was a lively affair that ended only when darkness fell.

But, one final surprise was in store for me that night. As I watched our unorthodox group of golfers make their way back to the parking lot, the automatic sprinkler system suddenly turned on. Huge plumes of water shot forty feet into the air from sprinkler heads all around us. And— of course—the counselors immediately wheeled their happily shrieking campers directly into the huge fountains of water, rather than retreating from them. After about fifteen minutes in this improvised water park, reminiscent of kids dancing around broken fire hydrants in the summer in New York City, Jabberwocky's drenched but happy golfers boarded the bus and vans and headed back to Camp, exuberant howls and laughter echoing in their wake.

I stayed behind to clean up and was horrified to see an impressive variety of punctures and tread marks in the formerly pristine practice green. I did my best to repair the divots and gashes, but real damage had been done. Let's just say that members of golf clubs can be finicky about the maintenance of their greens and fairways and I feared that, after this little escapade, I could expect to catch some serious flack. The next day, at lunch in the main cabin at Camp, the cook yelled to me over the din and said that I had a phone call.

"Who is it?"

"It's the golf pro from Mink Meadows."

"Shoot!"

I had been in a state of nervous denial all day. With the sinking feeling of being called into the principal's office, I walked into the kitchen and picked up the phone. "Hi, it's Doctor Steve. I'm really sorry about the ..."

He cut me off before I could finish the sentence.

"Some of the members contacted me today, and they all said the same thing."

Damn!

"Having Camp Jabberwocky as our guest at Mink Meadows was ..."

Shit!

"One of the best things that's happened to this club in a helluva long time. They want to know when you can bring the campers back again."

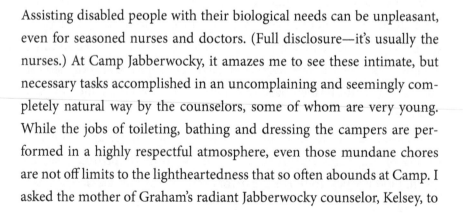

Assisting disabled people with their biological needs can be unpleasant, even for seasoned nurses and doctors. (Full disclosure—it's usually the nurses.) At Camp Jabberwocky, it amazes me to see these intimate, but necessary tasks accomplished in an uncomplaining and seemingly completely natural way by the counselors, some of whom are very young. While the jobs of toileting, bathing and dressing the campers are performed in a highly respectful atmosphere, even those mundane chores are not off limits to the lightheartedness that so often abounds at Camp. I asked the mother of Graham's radiant Jabberwocky counselor, Kelsey, to remind me of an incident at Camp that had made a lasting impression on her a number of years ago. Here is her reply:

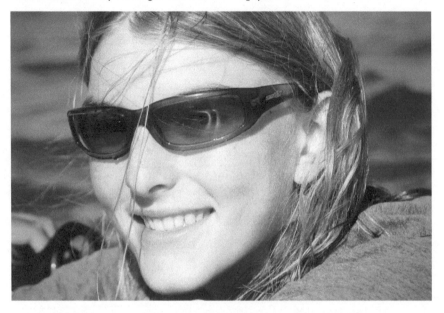

Kelsey

"Hi Steve,

Yes, I remember it well. I felt as though I had stumbled upon a moment of such love, compassion and humanity.

This was Kelsey's first full summer as a counselor. I believe she was seventeen. She was a camp groupie for a number of years prior to that. As a novice, I remember hoping she would be assigned a camper who was fairly uncomplicated—maybe one of the adults with Down Syndrome. When she learned she was assigned Graham, she called me with pure excitement in her voice, her confidence boosted by her selection as his counselor—Graham, the legendary, charming, nonverbal, medically fragile young man every counselor hoped to get.

I worried. She went through 'seizure training' in case he

should have an episode while in her care. He did, in the back of a van, when she was alone with him. She was clearly shaken and scared, but she did all the right things and they both got through it. She called to tell me what happened and her voice sounded different. It wasn't just that she was relieved he was alright. It was more that she was relieved that it was she who could be there for him, to offer empathy, comfort and support and to convey to him that she was truly 'there' for him—in the most present sense.

A few days later, I spontaneously dropped by to deliver a goodie bag of counselor supplies—candy, chocolate, snacks, shampoo, things the counselors never take time to go purchase for themselves because they didn't have any time. This was the only way I got to spend time with her in the summer. It was midafternoon and, after chatting with some of the happy campers, I was pointed in the direction of Kelsey and Graham's cabin. The door was ajar, and I entered a tidy little enclave of bunk beds, wheelchairs and improvised bug screens.

I heard splashing and giggling coming from the bathroom. Not knowing what I would find, I tentatively pressed open the door, and there I saw a naked Graham lying in a bathtub, his body cradled between Kelsey's legs as she sat behind him in a mismatched bikini. She was humming softly to him while lathering up his face for a shave. Her co-counselor was positioned outside the tub and gently wiped Graham's limbs with a soapy sponge. Startled by this raw, revealing moment, I took a moment to collect myself, with tears welling in my eyes. Using humor to diffuse the poignancy of what I was seeing, I said 'Hey, Graham ... look at you being bathed by two hot girls! You are the man.' He tilted his head back toward me, looked me in the eye—and let out a full-body squeal of delight.

Graham affected everyone lucky enough to spend time with him. After that summer, I remember thinking—as Kelsey was embarking on her college search—that it really doesn't matter what she achieves in life. I already know who she is. That was a gift of revelation Graham helped provide.

Love,

Corinne"

We were *all* invited. The entire eclectic Jabberwocky family with its kaleidoscopic spectrum of abilities and disabilities. The whole madcap collection of individuals from wildly different backgrounds—*all of us.* The pleasure of our company was requested! We were cordially invited! To our wonder and delight, Camp Jabberwocky was about to participate in that most joyous of summer celebrations: a wedding!

This marriage ceremony would be particularly poignant, because Jonathan Wolf and Mandy Adams were two of our own. Destined for careers in teaching and advocacy for the homeless, the couple had met at Camp as counselors several years earlier and fallen in love. Their families loved the Vineyard and were longtime Jabberwocky supporters. On an island known for gala events, this wedding promised to be the most romantic and magnificent social happening of the summer. Side-by-side with some well-heeled summer residents and visitors, we were all going to be part of it. Indeed, the wedding party itself, the bridesmaids and groomsmen, was to feature a sprinkling of campers and counselors.

There are elegant venues on Martha's Vineyard available for prominent social occasions, including yacht clubs and country clubs, but Jonathan and Mandy wanted their ceremony to be held on the campus of

Camp Jabberwocky. Shortly after we all arrived at Camp that summer, a big tent appeared in the field at the back of the property decorated with huge yellow and blue ribbons and vibrant bouquets of the island's signature flowers, blue hydrangeas. Anticipation was intense as the special day approached, just a few days after the start of Camp.

On the morning of the wedding, the Jabberwocky counselors, joyful young people of imagination and kindness, scrubbed and coiffed their campers until they nearly sparkled. Elegant finery from the "costume cabin" in the basement of Camp's theater replaced funky shorts and T-shirts. Two by two, the pairs of counselors and campers arrived for the ceremony, many approaching the tent in walkers and wheelchairs.

Under a dappled canopy of scrub oaks, I walked behind my son's wheelchair as his counselor pushed him along. A musician was seated near an improvised altar, playing the guitar and quietly singing "What a Wonderful World." My heart was full as I reflected on the choice made by the bride and groom to be married in that special place, a place defined by friendship, mutual support and love.

As the wedding congregation proceeded along the path to the big field, steeped in the sense of quiet reverence that surrounds a wedding, we witnessed a perfectly timed example of Camp Jabberwocky's playful *irreverence*. Someone had posted a handcrafted message on a tree for Mandy and Jonathan to see: "Turn back now!"

At the ceremony, Graham was at one end of an arc of wheelchairs to the right of the wedding party. I sat in the grass next to him, rested my arm on his and experienced the service at his side. I could not remember feeling the way I did in those moments ever before in my life. And yet it would not have been Camp Jabberwocky if the service had not been punctuated by laughter. A whimsical interlude was provided by our Camp directors that year, JoJo and Arthur, when they stood up and recited the Jabberwocky poem with zest and theatricality:

"The Jabberwocky with eyes of flame
Came whiffling through the tulgey wood
And burbled as it came!"

Moments later, under a beautiful chuppah, the symbolic tapestry that forms a protective wedding "canopy" over the bride and groom, Rabbi Rachel Cowan, who led the ceremony, spoke to Mandy and Jonathan about Camp Jabberwocky:

> "Here you are, surrounded and blessed by God's presence, open to everyone coming into your life. Chance, randomness and destiny have come together in this moment. This is where your love grows deep. This is where you feel deeply at home. This is where you overcome fears, take risks and grow. This is where you need a tremendous sense of humor! This is where you give and receive support. This is where you can be exactly who you are. This is where you trust your instincts and know you make a difference. This is where your hearts have no walls."

In the exquisite moments that followed, family, friends, campers and volunteers bore witness as the couple exchanged wedding vows. On the most important day of their lives, Mandy and Jonathan chose to include all of Camp Jabberwocky. They wanted us to know that the God blessing their marriage loves all of us, unconditionally.

There is a yurt at Camp nestled unobtrusively in the scrub oak woods that shelter the campus. Its circular structure is derived from the dwellings of Central Asian nomads. The round shape deflects the wind, although extreme weather conditions are uncommon in that protected part of the island in the summer. The yurt at Camp is open on the sides, providing the freeing sense of being outdoors, while still being covered by a roof. The idea for a yurt arose when Gillian, Hellcat's daughter, and our first camp director, wanted to create a circular area for dance. She found out about a man from Maine named Bill Copperthwaite who builds yurts and believes in living simply, thinking things through and working together. A collaboration was born, and before long, Camp Jabberwocky had its yurt.

A variety of relatively meditative activities takes place there during Camp. Classes in the yurt tend to be reflective, even spiritual, in nature and offer a respite from the generally frenetic events going on elsewhere around the campus. Graham was in the yurt one day with a small group led by Maggie and Michelle, his joyful and soulful counselors that year. They sensed that Graham wanted to show off his walking skills. Supported by someone strong, Graham could occasionally take small steps. His feet would get tangled, but with the right nudging and support, he could painstakingly move one frail leg and then the other. His mother was masterful at helping him to "walk" this way, and she encouraged the rest of us to work at it. Without assistance, Graham could not even stand, but with help, short bursts of laborious efforts to walk were possible for him, at least on those occasions when he was comfortable in his body.

Giving campers a chance to show off the skill of walking is a central theme at Camp. At mealtime, campers who are able to do it, even taking just a step or two while leaning heavily on their counselors, are given the chance to enter the main cabin on their own two feet, an effort always rewarded by hearty cheers. For camper and counselor, this plodding into the main cabin is typically a painstaking and slow process. Yet, even though everyone inside is hungry, the entire camp family waits patiently for those who want to give it a try, to "walk" into the dining area on their own two feet.

Maggie and Michelle had actually never seen Graham really try to walk. For him, taking even a few steps with assistance took immense concentration and effort. For his aides elsewhere, it was often easier to simply not bother with it, leaving him to sit all day in his wheelchair. However, on this particular July day, spurred on by the combined strength and encouragement of Maggie and Michelle, Graham improbably walked around the entire perimeter of the yurt, an odyssey that took some fifteen minutes and required enormous effort and focus by all three. The counselors were astonished. It was a "Jabberwocky moment," one of the surprising and thrilling epiphanies that occur at Camp with some regularity. Upon completing his loop around the circumference of the yurt, an effort perhaps like someone else running a marathon, Graham looked proudly at Maggie and Michelle. And then he erupted in silly, unrestrained laughter that seemed to convulse his entire being.

When Michelle related the story to me later, she said simply:

"That was the best moment of my life."

One of Graham's best friends at Camp Jabberwocky was Virginia Hackney. Long a beloved personage on the Vineyard, Virginia enjoyed a kind of hybrid role at Camp, not quite a camper and not exactly a counselor. By the time we met her, she was about forty years old and had short, graying hair that emerged in an unpredictable tangle from the sides of a baseball cap. She was free to come and go as she pleased, and she divided her time between Camp and her many other passions on the island. Although Virginia was said to have a "mental handicap," she was sharper than most people in many ways, including having a memory that was sometimes spooky.

Whatever she was doing, Virginia lived every day exuberantly, starting with breakfast at the famous Black Dog Tavern in Vineyard Haven.
From a table that was permanently reserved for her, she held court with
the servers and cooks who loved to dote on her. After breakfast she
would appear at Camp on the Trek bike that symbolized her fierce sense
of independence, spend a few hours and then ride off to figure skating
practice, choir practice at the Grace Church or rehearsals at the Vineyard
Playhouse, where she loved being on stage. Her enthusiasm, irreverent
humor and kindness were uniquely endearing and the island community
embraced Virginia. At Seasons, a pub in Oak Bluffs, Virginia was noto-
rious for her karaoke performances of Madonna's "Material Girl," to the
delight of a multitude of gleeful friends.

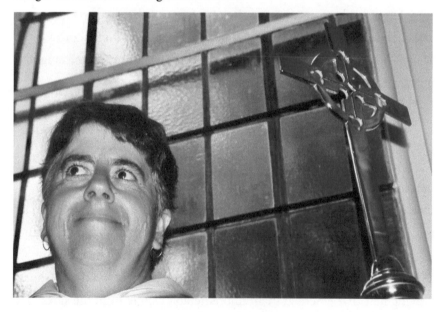

Virginia at Grace Church

Virginia was much loved during her life and the battle she waged
bravely with pancreatic cancer, supported by her adoring family and
her legion of "fans," as her family called us. I visited Virginia on a few

occasions when she was an inpatient at MGH for treatment. The illness never dimmed her radiant spirit. When I would say goodbye from the door of her hospital room, she offered me the same mischievous admonition she gave to all her friends:

"Behave!"

There was a telling incident that involved Virginia one Sunday at Grace Church in Vineyard Haven, where she was a fixture in the choir. A camper from Jabberwocky had been invited to sing a solo part in a hymn, but, when the time came to stand up in front of the congregation, she developed stage fright and froze. The congregation held its collective breath for a few agonizing moments until someone popped out from the choir pews, grabbed the camper's hand and sang the hymn with her as if nothing had happened. That person was Virginia.

Virginia adored Graham and never failed to compliment him on how handsome he was. Each year she bought him a present, typically a trendy Black Dog T-shirt. Without fail, Graham could count on receiving a gift adorned with the famous Labrador retriever logo before leaving Camp. When Virginia became ill, however, for the first time in our experience, a camp session passed without Graham seeing his old friend. Consumed by the frenetic pace of camp, we didn't give Virginia's absence too much thought until a few weeks later, back at home, a package arrived from the Vineyard. A beautiful royal blue T-shirt from the Black Dog. We had heard by then about Virginia's cancer and reached her by phone at the condo where she still lived independently on Main Street in Vineyard Haven.

"Virginia, we are awfully sorry to hear about your diagnosis. How are you doing?"

"Don't worry about me, I'm doing just fine. How did Graham like his T-shirt?"

A spirited fall tradition that Graham and I started was taking a group from Camp Jabberwocky to a Harvard football game in the storied ivy-covered stadium on Soldier's Field Road across the Charles River from Cambridge. Our friend from Salem, Dr. Don Sadoski, carefully planned the first event for us, which was preceded by a lively tailgate party hosted by his wife, Darlene and their extended family. Don played football at Harvard and still loyally supports the team. He keeps an eye out for exceptional student athletes from the towns north of Boston who might be candidates for the school and its teams. But I sensed that Don also recognized something uncommon in Graham.

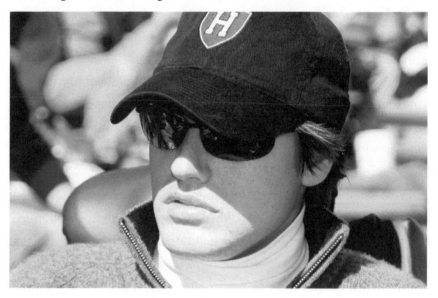

Graham at Harvard Stadium

The accessible area at Harvard Stadium happens to be in the very front row. From that choice spot, the Harvard players and cheerleaders are just a few feet in front of us, while the Harvard student section is right behind us. If you turn around from the front row and look up into the stands, you see hundreds of students who are literally among the most gifted and motivated young people in the world, relaxing, however briefly, on a crisp fall Saturday in New England. As a preceptor in the Harvard Medical School's teaching programs, I have interacted with scores of those amazing young people. They are smart *and* they are kind, exactly the traits you might hope to find in a physician—or anyone else. They uniformly understand the responsibility of *noblesse oblige*, the ancient notion that, from those to whom much has been given, much should be expected.

Of course, to be accepted at Harvard, or any other elite school, is no small feat these days. It may not even be enough to be a high school valedictorian with perfect SAT scores and a lengthy track record of public service. The kids up in those ancient concrete bleachers are part of a very rarified group.

Graham and his handicapped mates in the front row appeared to stand in sharp contrast to that elite group. More accurately, they *sat* in sharp contrast in their wheelchairs. But, as the years passed, I found myself wondering about the apparent disparity. And was it really so striking? What, in fact, if Graham applied to an elite college? A young man who could not read or write was surely not "Harvard material." Unable to communicate conventionally and dependent on others for everything, what could Graham offer an Ivy League university? I pondered that, glancing back and forth from our group to the wunderkinds behind us.

Although his body was maddeningly uncooperative, Graham was undeniably intelligent. He possessed an understanding that was sensed by his caregivers in the nuances of his expressions and vocalizations. He was absolutely honest. He was free of prejudice. He did his best every day. He was a loyal friend. He was loving, kind and fun. And he personified decency. His radiant spirit inspired others.

I had always sensed that our friend, Doctor Don Sadoski, recognized something special in Graham. Could it have been "Harvard material?"

4

BAD THINGS, GOOD PEOPLE

Graham became critically ill with a mysterious illness when he was twelve, and we spent three harrowing months in the dead of winter at Children's Hospital in Boston. Children's is one of the triumphant institutions of our civilization, a place where extraordinarily bright and compassionate people do everything in their power to assist any child in distress, regardless of means or background, twenty-four hours a day, 365 days a year. But, Graham had even those exceptional nurses and doctors stumped. He was suffering from an elusive type of encephalitis, an inflammation of the brain, that no medication could relieve, with fevers up to 105 degrees, stupor, persistent grand mal seizures and abject exhaustion. As Graham neared death, we grew desperate, seemingly out of options.

In the lobby of the famous hospital were huge oil paintings of world-renowned emeritus Harvard pediatricians in white jackets and bow ties. We succeeded in coaxing one or two, long retired, to come in and try to assist us. But even they could not explain Graham's illness or suggest an effective treatment. In what can be an ominous development—meaning the medical team is fearing the worst—one of the hospital's kind chaplains came to see us to offer prayer and counseling. She gave us a copy of Rabbi

Harold Kushner's *When Bad Things Happen to Good People,* among other readings that were intended to provide even a little comfort to parents facing the imminent possibility of losing a child. Rabbi Kushner knew his subject from the perspective of profound personal pain. His own son, Aaron, had died at about Graham's age.

Essentially, the theological conundrum that Rabbi Kushner explores in the book is whether God can be good *and* omnipotent. If God is both good *and* in control of everything, then unspeakable tragedies, like the Holocaust, pandemics and disasters, would never happen. Accordingly, if God is good, God cannot also be in control. I understood Kushner's conclusion to mean that God is present in the love that we experience in our lives and, especially in the kindness we receive in times of crisis. But God does not want bad things to happen to children or anyone else. During the long illness, Graham received well wishes from old and new friends. After a time, the previously barren walls of his ICU room became essentially covered with overlapping get well cards. The room began to feel like a cave decorated with a kaleidoscopic mosaic made from messages of love.

Still, he remained critically ill.

In our darkest hour, when Graham was essentially comatose, Cynthia cradled him and asked him if he wanted to stay or if it was his time to let go. If he was ready to go, we would try to allow that unthinkable thing to happen, knowing it would be the most horrific decision we would ever make. I watched Cynthia hold him close, her face pressed against his, and ask him to tell us what he wanted to do.

"You can go, Bud, if you need to. But you have to show us a sign. We will honor whatever decision you make, no matter how painful it is for us."

Graham's ICU room featured the usual cacophonous jumble of monitors and medical gadgets on poles, with no windows to the outside world. Yet, as Cynthia cradled her son, something curious happened. We became aware of a warm breeze and a current of air that set the scores of cards subtly rippling in a pattern that circled the room. It was reminiscent of the rhythmic "wave" that the 37,000 baseball fans at Fenway Park, just down Brookline Avenue from the hospital, create in a playful sequence at every Red Sox home game. If there was a vent of some kind in the room that could explain that breeze, we hadn't noticed it before. We chose a different interpretation. Cynthia had asked our son for a sign and that warm breeze was his answer: Graham did not want to go!

And, miraculously—there was no other word for it—as a few purple crocuses and yellow daffodils emerged from the dirty snow outside the hospital, Graham got just a little better. There were fewer pained movements and less grimacing. His fever slowly resolved. It would be a long time before he was his old self again, but, against the better judgment of some of his caregivers, we made a decision and took Graham home. He would remain frail and restless for many months more.

But Graham had survived.

During Graham's nightmarish illness at Children's Hospital, Cynthia and I reached a breaking point. In those dreadful days and nights, we were barely hanging on emotionally. Thankfully, a stream of visitors brought us much-needed strength and comfort. According to Rabbi Kushner, God's presence was manifest at a time like that in the support of loving people. We also, however, experienced disappointment. People we would have expected to be there for us simply never came or called. Was it the closeness of death that kept them away? Or, was it not knowing how to act around a family with a disability? Cynthia and I struggled to understand and forgive those people. Wandering the quiet hospital floors late at night, I thought of a phrase from the poignant ballad "I Don't Know Why" by Shawn Colvin: "They're not trying to cause you pain. They're just afraid of loving you." At Children's Hospital, Cynthia, Graham and I had to accept that there might be reasons why some otherwise fine people had a hard time dealing with a situation like ours.

The kids who grew up with Graham, however, were not at all afraid to love him. Daria Pecorella, a dark-haired beauty of nine or ten, was one. She visited him regularly and hovered around the head of his bed, talking nonstop and stroking his satiny hair. During one of those visits, a nurse came in to start an IV.

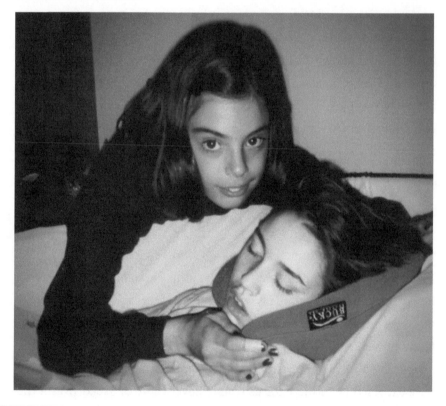

Daria with Graham

"Deary, I have to do something with Graham now that might be uncomfortable. Would you step out for a minute?"

"No, I'd prefer to stay right here with my friend, thank you."

And she stayed right there.

While we received scores of comforting visits from family and friends, like Daria and her brother Alex, the kindness of people we barely knew was surprising and life-giving. Jim Yelsits was a pharmaceutical executive who had visited my office in Boston a number of times to talk to our clinical staff about the new medications his company was developing. He and I had quickly become friendly on the level of professional acquaintances, but we didn't know each other outside the setting of my office. The first Sunday after Graham was admitted to Children's, a nurse stuck her head in his room and announced that we had visitors. Jim and his radiant wife, Karen, walked in bearing cut flowers, palms from their church and a completely natural aura of good will. With no apprehension or hesitation, they took Graham's hand and began to talk to him. They engaged him instantly in an upbeat, playful way. The couple brought all three of us a feeling of solidarity, and it is not hyperbole to say that they filled Graham's room with love that day.

We didn't really know Jim and Karen at all, but they had driven a considerable distance to meet Graham and to lend the three of us their spiritual support. Both of them saw straight through Graham's disability and into the remarkable boy inside. They visited regularly, typically on Sundays, until we made it home from the hospital. A few weeks later, when Graham was feeling better, we were guests in Jim and Karen's home and were able to tell them how just how much their kindness had meant to us.

5

CROTCHED MOUNTAIN

"We love the things we love for what they are."
—Robert Frost

As you enter New Hampshire on the highway from Massachu-setts, you can see Crotched Mountain on the horizon with its twin north-facing peaks and its flatter plateau to the south. That scenic southern ridge provides the protected, pastoral setting for the Crotched Mountain School and Rehabilitation Center, Graham's alma mater and his weekday home between the ages of twelve and twenty-two. Cynthia and I had decided that Graham needed the support and services that Crotched offered after his harrowing illness. En route to spending occasional weekends there with Graham (more often he came home to Massachusetts), I always marveled at that first, almost ethereal glimpse of the mountain that was frequently cloaked in mist. Graham was up there in that lofty place that had been inspired by the belief that people with disabilities deserve the same opportunities to learn and seek their potential as everyone else.

Founded in 1953 (curiously, the same year as Camp Jabberwocky), caring initially for children with polio and deafness, Crotched Mountain's school and rehabilitation clinics have always served the needs of vulnerable children and adults with significant medical and cognitive challenges; people who might not receive optimal help in their own communities. I was amazed, from the time of our first interview there, that such a place existed at all in times of economic austerity and, further, that it was situated in one of the most breathtaking settings in all of New England. My drive on winding country roads passed marshes and dairy farms until I could feel the Jeep laboring up the final steep pitch along the side of Crotched Mountain. Suddenly, out of a thick pine forest, the campus would appear and I would park excitedly at Graham's dorm some 2,000 feet above sea level.

I wondered if the founder of Crotched Mountain had placed the school and hospital on the highest spot he could find, as a metaphor for the arduous climb his clients would need to complete in order to achieve their dreams. I wondered, too, if Harry Gregg, the philanthropist and inspired founder of the center, felt that in a mystical place with a panoramic view of the world below, the foundation's humanitarian mission could more easily flourish. Insulated from the commercial and cultural noise of the bustling towns and cities below, there was nothing on that beautiful plateau above Greenfield that could disturb the center's mission.

After emotional weekend visits with Graham in a country that resonated with the imagery of Robert Frost, it was difficult to leave him and descend the mountain. The world below seemed increasingly characterized by discord and superficiality. Leaving that summit meant leaving a kind of sanctuary. I had a melancholy feeling whenever I left. While Graham clearly needed the resources of Crotched Mountain, I still wished that he could just come home with me and attend a regular school. But my unhappy feeling was offset by a sense of gratitude that a place like Crotched even exists and that Graham was fortunate enough to be part of it.

When Harry Gregg founded the facility in 1953, he wrote that he was so excited that he couldn't sleep at night, imagining all the possibilities that lay ahead to make the future brighter for people with disabilities. Happily, the spiritual descendants of Harry Gregg can be found at Crotched Mountain today, caring passionately for children and adults with a variety of challenges.

In a pivotal stroke of good fortune, the effervescent Lisa Prescott was assigned to be Graham's licensed nursing assistant (LNA) at Crotched Mountain when he arrived there at age twelve. An LNA is a skilled, full-time caregiver who helps a disabled person with his "activities of daily living," including personal care, attending school and therapy sessions, and anything else that comes up in the course of a day. Lisa had worked in that capacity with many youngsters at Crotched in the years before her new protege appeared. At the time of Graham's arrival, he was emerging from the horrific illness that had trapped him at Children's Hospital for three months. Lisa's caring presence and willingness to go above and beyond contributed immensely to his recovery in the challenging months that followed. Her commitment to her new client was thoroughly professional, but a heartfelt, personal connection developed between the two almost instantly.

From her very first days with Graham, Lisa resolved that he would enjoy the best possible quality of life during his time at Crotched Mountain. That meant having fun together, in addition to getting the most out of school and therapy. The friendship that began that summer deepened steadily over the next decade.

Lisa grew up in rural New England, but she was not unsophisticated. The svelte strawberry blonde took great pride in the way both she and Graham looked. Cynthia and I always knew that our son's grooming and hygiene were impeccable. Knowing that Lisa was there as Graham's advocate and confidante was a powerful gift. It was especially delightful to know that the two spent parts of every day laughing together.

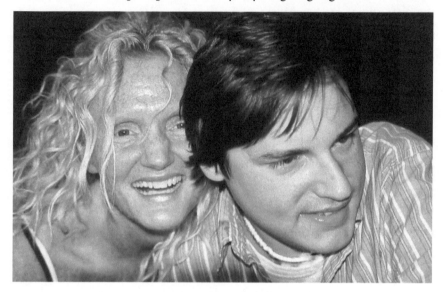

Graham and Lisa

Lisa frequently came down from New Hampshire over the years to help Cynthia and me with Graham when he was home in Massachusetts. When Graham was a little older, Lisa joined us for our "spring break" vacations in the Caribbean, which would not have been possible without her help. Those special weeks became an annual high point for us and a reward for surviving the long New England winter. Our tropical trips were portals to adventure that many people would have considered off-limits to someone like Graham. Our debt to Lisa is immeasurable.

With her permission, here is part of a remembrance that she shared with us after Graham passed away:

> "Graham Gardner was a gift I didn't know I would have for only
> a limited time. He brought me complete happiness. To me, he

was perfect. He was grateful for every small thing I did for him. He appreciated me for who I was. He loved me for who I was. He never took anything I did for him for granted. He always tried to greet me with his radiant smile and amazing presence. And even when he was having a hard day, and he was not able to greet me with that smile, he would just look at me, and I knew he was happy to see me. We depended on each other. He needed me to help him with all aspects of life. And he helped me to appreciate life itself."

When I visited Graham for the weekend at Crotched Mountain, I usually found him waiting for me with his aide near the nursing station of the Hayden Building on a Saturday morning. Hayden was Graham's dormitory, but it also served as a small children's hospital for kids with head injuries and other neurological issues. There was usually a pleasant hustle and bustle around the nursing station and, after my ninety-minute drive, I couldn't wait to burst through the doors of Hayden, turn the corner and lay eyes on my gorgeous son. I would usually find him sitting patiently in the middle of a group of kids in wheelchairs, interacting in the relaxed atmosphere of the weekend with some aides and family members of a few dorm mates.

Of course, I would bend down and greet Graham effusively. It was impossible not to do so! But sometimes his immediate response to me was muted. While I wondered if it was because we were in a public area, I sometimes felt a pang of disappointment when he did not instantly greet me with the same enthusiasm I showed. After saying hello to the staff, I would wheel Graham down to his sunny room at the end of the corridor with its view of the north peak of Crotched Mountain. After closing the door, I would face him squarely, kneel down to his eye level, grab his shoulders and tell him how happy it made me to know that he was my son and that we would be together for a whole weekend.

After a few seconds, a slight tremor would appear in his arms. Moments later, the tremor would expand into an explosive contraction of Graham's whole body, accompanied by a goofy ear-to-ear smile and a shriek of joy as he looked straight into my eyes. It simply took Graham a while to process stimuli and to react to them. His neurons worked at their own pace. The teachers, therapists, camp counselors and friends who knew him well learned to slow things down and give his nervous system a chance to work. Lisa was an expert at this and always allowed Graham extra time to respond to questions. Donna Chadwick, his music therapist at Crotched, was masterfully patient with him and discovered unique surprises as a result. And for his father, the reward for awaiting Graham's delayed Saturday morning greetings in his room at Crotched Mountain were moments of nothing less than pure joy.

In medical school, we were taught about an emotion called "anticipatory grief." It refers to the idea that you can actually grieve about something before it happens, when you know that what is about to happen will likely make you miserable. The concept crystallized for me one summer day while kayaking with Graham at Sunset Lake below Crotched Mountain, when I found myself missing him—even though we were still together! The emotion was silly, but I couldn't deny it. On visits to Crotched Mountain, I would actually start to miss Graham sometime on Saturday, fully aware that we had most of the weekend ahead of us. I would miss him even more on Sunday morning, despite knowing that we were going to be together all day. I missed Graham in the middle of vacation weeks, fully aware that he wouldn't have to return to school for five days and that we would be together all that time.

In our particular manner, Graham and I communicated about that idiotic emotion of mine and what it meant, psychologically. Maybe I just hated the idea of not being with him—all the time. He would listen to my ruminations and respond with a sly smile. Often, when we communicated, Graham would also use his voice, making sounds that fell short of distinct words. His vocalizations, however, had intonation and emotional power. They frequently seemed to have a subject, a verb and an object. Those of us who loved him usually knew exactly what he meant.

Graham and I talked to each other throughout our weekends at Crotched, and it was clear to me that my son grasped every nuance of those "conversations." My anticipatory grief was a recurring theme and became a kind of inside joke between us. I could usually get him to chuckle by insisting that one way you know you really love someone is that you miss him terribly. Even while you're still with him.

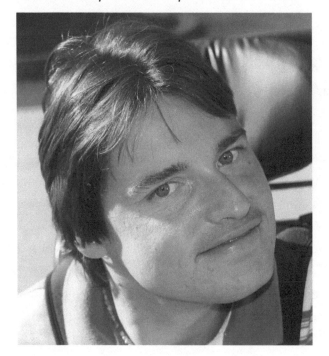

Sadly, when I was growing up, it was not uncommon to hear someone like Graham referred to as a "retard." I recall my own friends in grade school saying cruel things about a classmate with polio. Perhaps surprisingly, I don't believe that Cynthia and I ever heard unkind words spoken about our son, although it's possible that we were just naive.

To his music therapist at Crotched Mountain, Donna Chadwick, Graham was about as far from being mentally retarded as a human being can be. In a remembrance, she described him in terms that surprised even us, Graham's adoring parents. Coming from one of the most erudite, soulful and compassionate people we had ever met, hers was a stunning description of a boy who never spoke, at least conventionally:

> "Let me tell you about Graham the musician. He put maximum physical and emotional effort into music-making. He found freedom and euphoria in music. With his right hand, Graham played chimes, bells and drums suspended from the ceiling. He reached to play electronic keyboard keys while I improvised songs and we played together.
>
> Receptively, he absorbed music. He vocalized full throttle without words. With his hands, he pressed a mechanical voice simulation switch on which lyrics were recorded. He inserted those words, a little like karaoke, while I played the song accompaniment on piano or guitar. The precision with which Graham achieved motor control and his eager practice to supply these musical phrases at just the right time indicated his gift of a sensitive musical intelligence.
>
> In my decades as a therapist credentialed in three disciplines, I have never met anyone as exquisite as Graham Gardner.

He is one of the most influential people I have ever known. Beyond his physical beauty, his enormous striving, his magnetic personality, his tender gestures like holding hands, Graham lived a directed and purposeful life. He taught, collaborated, inspired, expressed, created.

Graham's intelligence was evident. We wrote songs together, using the technique of guided composition, which helps individuals who don't communicate with words to decide upon song topics, lyrics and accompaniment.

Graham possessed a knowing. Simply being in his presence was elevating. Graham was pure, authentic, trusting and loving. He accepted his reality, lived in the present moment, reveled in relationships and released radiance all around him. Graham personified joy and he lived love. And love is eternal.

According to current teachings, Graham was a spiritual master."

During Graham's decade as a residential student at Crotched Mountain, Cynthia would usually drive up to southern New Hampshire from the Boston area and pick him up on Fridays, so we could have him in our homes for the weekend in Marblehead and Salem. Cynthia and I both came to know every twist and turn on the ninety-minute drive to the school, and couldn't wait to lay our hands on the lad after not seeing him for several days. It was wonderful to have Graham at our homes, but I also enjoyed going up to the school and spending occasional weekends with Graham there. For one thing, it was a chance to give his mom a rare weekend to herself. It was also interesting to spend time with the people who took such great care of Graham and an opportunity to get to know some of his classmates and their families.

There were marvelous things for Graham and me to do in that magnificent White Mountain region of New Hampshire. We learned to paddle
in one of the school's kayaks on Sunset Lake. We took long walks on the
wooded trails around the campus, occasionally spotting white-tailed
deer. We swam in the heated therapy pool. We bounced basketballs in
the quiet gym. But the best part of those weekends was simply spending
time together. *Being* together. Slowing down from the rapid pace of the
week and savoring unhurried moments—together.

On one wall of Graham's room hung a hand-calligraphed copy of Rudyard Kipling's poem "If" that had been a gift to me from my mother years
before. I often read it aloud to Graham to remind him of how proud he
made his mother and me, dealing bravely with epilepsy and many other
challenges:

> "If you can force your heart and nerve and sinew
> To serve your turn long after they are gone
> And so hold on when there is nothing in you
> Except the will which says to them: 'Hold on …'
> You'll be a man, my son."

From Graham's dorm room, we watched the seasons change on the
summit of the mountain. We took naps side by side in his single bed,
cramped but content. We watched sports on TV. And sometimes Graham
would listen attentively as I read aloud some poems by Robert Frost.

Crotched Mountain is in the Monadnock region, the heart of pastoral
New Hampshire that is the setting for many of Frost's poems. The farms,
stone walls and massive stands of pines and birch in that part of the state
are the backdrop for his most famous works. The poet was a farmer at
one time in nearby Derry. Graham and I had an illustrated volume that
grouped the poems according to the season. We could read a poem aloud

and, later, on our walks, experience bucolic scenes nearly identical to those we had just read about.

In winter, we bundled up and braved the winds on the mountain top, dry snow crunching under the big wheels of Graham's "jogger." Sometimes we stopped to consider the warm glow from windows, like the narrator in Frost's winter poems, wondering what the people inside were doing.

In the spring, we looked for the first crocuses, celebrated the arrival of the robins and waited for the last patches of dirty snow to melt. We saw saplings bent over from the weight of winter ice, but still alive and determined to grow strong again, like the patients in the Crotched Mountain Hospital who were recovering from brain injuries.

In summer, we swam in the lake, visited local ice cream stands with Lisa and savored the long, lazy days without having to bundle up in layers of heavy clothing.

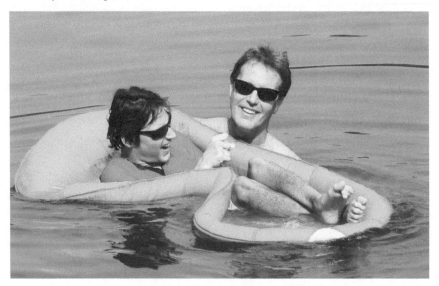

Sunset Lake

In the fall, we went apple picking, sensing with mixed emotions the distinct crispness in the air that signals the end of another cycle of life in New England. As the birch groves around the mountain turned yellow, we looked for new paths in the woods around the campus to explore. It was natural at that time of year for us to be drawn to Frost's most famous fall poem, "The Road Not Taken," about two roads diverging in a yellow wood and how taking the one "less traveled" changed the life of the narrator. Every September, I would ask Graham if I should read that poem and his reaction always told me that he wanted to hear it. Our own path in life was different than what we might have predicted, due to Graham's disability. As Frost famously observed, "way leads on to way," and I knew that we would not be traveling conventional roads in the future.

The path we were on, along with Graham's mom, was unexpected, but it was defined by our own set of values. We were on a road less traveled, but we were traveling it together, and our path was defined entirely by love. And that has made all the difference.

On his graduation day, after nearly a decade at Crotched Mountain, Graham wore a royal blue cap and gown before we said emotional thank yous and goodbyes and descended the mountain for the final time.

6

BEING TOGETHER

Jabberwocky owns a small house a short distance down Greenwood Avenue from the main fourteen-acre Camp property. Like all the other Camp buildings, it was given a name from the famous poem and became known as *Whiffling*. Historically, the camp doctor and other volunteers were eligible to use the house during their time at Camp. I typically shared the modest home with my friends, the effervescent Ho family. Mike and Kim and their three decidedly different daughters, Gabrielle, Madeline and Larissa were usually there with me at the beginning of the first Camp session of the summer. Never having had sisters or daughters, it was a treat for me to be under the same roof with that trio of spirited girls, even though Larissa sometimes was ready to start her day at about the same time as a flock of wild turkeys started theirs, noisily squawking in our back yard around dawn.

I was allowed to take Graham for lunch with me at Whiffling, a special privilege that I negotiated with Gillian Butchman, our camp director. Our arrangement was an exception to the Jabberwocky principle that discourages parental involvement during camp sessions. Families are expected to trust that Camp is fully capable of caring for their loved ones and to allow them to be immersed completely in the twenty-four-hour rhythms of life at Jabberwocky. Furthermore, Camp was founded, in part, with the goal of giving parents a respite. But Graham was attending Crotched Mountain during the week for much of the year. Happily for us, the camp director realized that his weeks on the Vineyard represented important bonding time for the two of us, even though it was also his coveted Jabberwocky time. Gillian's concession to let me take Graham down the street for lunch turned out to be a profound gift. The time we spent at Whiffling was exquisite, in surprising ways.

At the end of morning camp activities, I would collect my special friend and wheel him down the sandy blacktop of Greenwood Avenue. Roughing up his hair from behind and knowing that he was all mine for an hour or two filled me with happiness. Inside Whiffling, I would lie him down in the ground floor bedroom and give him a rest while I heated up the tasty lunches his mom had frozen for us before camp started. While feeding him those meals, I felt us both slow down from the sometimes dizzying pace of camp.

Lunch was followed by the brushing of teeth with Tom's Silly Strawberry toothpaste, a shave, facial moisturizer and a dash of Royall Mandarin cologne. Time permitting, we snuck in a quick nap before the counselors appeared and grabbed Graham for the afternoon activities.

Over the years, those lunch hours gave Graham and me time to develop an ever-deepening bond, simply being together in an atmosphere that was quiet and comfortable. Over lunch, we could communicate in our unique way about his progress at camp or listen to music and watch slide shows of the photographs I took every day.

While we were usually alone at lunch, we enjoyed the intermittent company of the Ho family and, occasionally, an unpredictable trickle of visitors. One day, a counselor named Adam somehow fell against a tree trunk and suffered what may have been a mild concussion. During lunch, we kept him on our couch for observation and intermittently quizzed him with the Bob Dylan lyrics he (and I!) knew by heart to see if he remained oriented. (He did.)

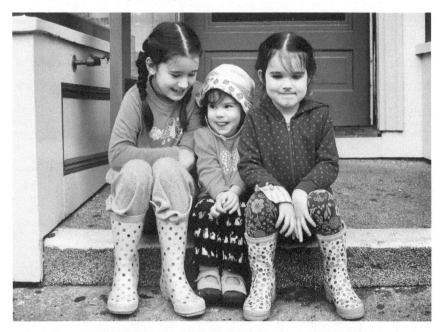

Whiffling housemates

Our hours at Whiffling were filled with the simplest kind of joy. Just being together was reassuring and life-giving. We were father and son, but also compadres for life and fellow members of a madcap family called Jabberwocky. When there was a thunderstorm and Camp's afternoon activities were delayed, we were given the bonus of extra time to relax together. On those occasions, we would lie side-by-side on my bed and listen to the rainfall.

Lisa and Cynthia took Graham to California for a vacation one year. They decided that swimming with the dolphins at Sea World might be an exciting experience for Graham and made the arrangements. Sea World requires that everyone who goes in the water must wear a wetsuit. Graham was normally patient and cooperative with his parents' grand ambitions for him. But, on this occasion, he just wasn't interested and let his two companions know it. Eventually, he came around and enjoyed the experience, but the adventure got off to a bad start. Lisa laughingly related the story as follows:

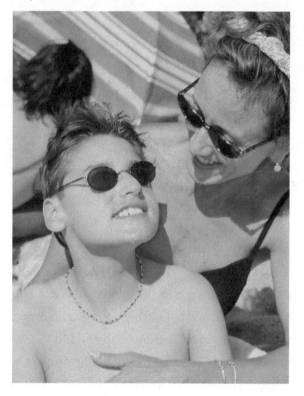

Cynthia and Graham readying for adventure

"Cynthia and I were laboring to get Graham into his wetsuit. You know how difficult that can be for yourself! There were no changing tables, so we had to put Graham on the floor. He was so uncooperative that he flopped around like a fish out of water. He yelled at us throughout the whole process, and it took us about thirty minutes to get the suit on him. When we were done, all three of us were exhausted.

Cynthia and I looked at him and asked 'Are you ready to swim with the dolphins?' He looked at us and, clear as day, he said, 'NO!'

Maybe you had to be there to see Graham's face, but it was hysterical to hear the vehemence in his voice.

Cynthia then looked at me and said, 'Next year we're going bird watching.'"

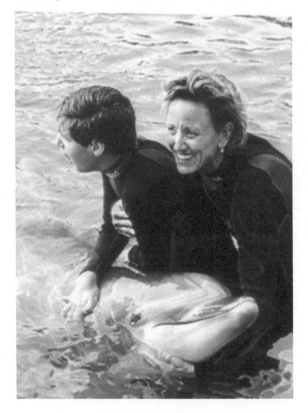

Perseverance pays off

During his time at Crotched Mountain, Graham and I discovered that we could paddle together on Sunset Lake in one of the school's kayaks. Gliding on the calm water gave us an exhilarating sense of freedom, and we decided to buy a boat of our own. We wanted a kayak that was inflatable with comfortable backrests. The only one available on the internet that fit our requirements was painted in "camouflage" greens and browns, apparently for the purpose of duck hunting. Neither Graham nor I owned a shotgun or any live ammunition, so hunting for food or sport was not in our destiny. But the kayak served our purposes perfectly.

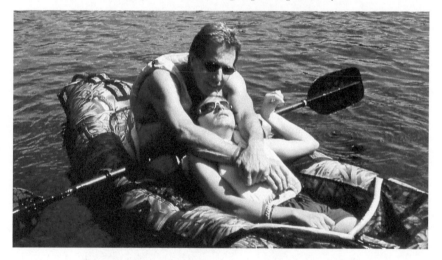

The forward seat was Graham's, and it had a soft but firm back support that he could lean against. I would sit or kneel behind him and paddle. It was virtually impossible to tip over. Besides the clear, smooth waters of Sunset Lake, we favored Winter Island in Salem, Riverhead Beach in Marblehead and the protected inner harbor of Vineyard Haven. Invariably, being on the water would calm Graham's nervous system, and I could actually see his muscles relaxing. On many occasions, the motion of the kayak and the rippling sounds of the water were so calming for Graham that he would fall completely asleep, sometimes within minutes of launching the boat.

On one of our outings, Graham's left arm repeatedly flexed back over his head in my direction in what I assumed was a kind of involuntary spasm. I noticed the same thing the next time we went out on a crisp fall day in Collins Cove, near our home in Salem. Graham's left arm arched back a number of times in my direction. We were approaching a cluster of moored boats near the mouth of the Danvers River when it hit me. Graham's movement was not a muscle spasm. It was *volitional*. Graham was literally reaching out to me. With his left arm, he was offering me a kind of "high five."

Graham was seeking my hand, as I had grasped his thousands of times. He was making a statement, albeit a nonverbal one. I wasn't completely sure, but I hoped he was telling me, "Dad, this is awesome fun! I love it out here," or "Dad, thank you. I know that you're proud of me. I'm proud of you, too," or "Dad, I know that you love me. I love you, too. But would you mind picking up the pace a little?"

As youngsters, my younger brother, Will, and I would hound our mom until she took us to Brigham's, the iconic chain of old-fashioned ice cream parlors in the Boston area. Brigham's was beloved in every New England home with children and served ice cream sundaes in metal dishes with abundant hot fudge and whipped cream. Their thick milk shakes, known in New England as "frappes," were served in immense Coca Cola glasses, with plenty left over in the frosty metal malt cup for you to refill your glass. Chocolate and vanilla were tasty, but coffee frappes became our all-time family favorite.

I hadn't thought about Brigham's for many years, until one summer at Camp Jabberwocky. It had started to bother me that Graham couldn't enjoy typical kids' treats, like pizza, popcorn and burgers. He just didn't have the motor control to chew those foods safely. He was a good sport about it and seemed content enough to eat the healthy meals his mom prepared. We chopped his food up in a processor and fed it to him bite by bite, a process that required patience all around. But it seemed unfair, at times, for the rest of us to be enjoying a lobster roll or fried clams while Graham was eating his veggie lasagna.

On a particularly glorious summer day, Graham and I were returning from an outing at State Beach with a small group of Jabberwocky campers and counselors jammed noisily into my Jeep Grand Cherokee. We had lifted Graham into the passenger seat so that he could ride shotgun. Our bunch was the overflow from the big Camp group riding in the Red Bus, the iconic vehicle so well known around the island. All of us, including Graham, had sand between the toes of our bare feet, salty skin and noses red from too much sun. Our bathing suits were a bit wet and itchy, but that offshoot of a day at the beach hardly bothered us as we sang along with tunes from the car radio. The windows were down and we were savoring the ocean breeze after a long day at the famous beach where parts of the movie *Jaws* were filmed.

When we slowed down to pass through the village of Oak Bluffs, I felt the Jeep being irresistibly drawn to Mad Martha's, the venerable ice cream parlor across from the old movie house. By custom, everyone from Camp was supposed to return to Vineyard Haven from the beach, so our pit stop was slightly unfair to the rest of the campers and counselors on the Red Bus who were not stopping at Mad Martha's. We took a quick poll, however, and decided that, if we were discreet, what the others didn't know wouldn't hurt them too much.

The crew ordered various ice cream treats and settled back in the Jeep to savor them. On a whim, I decided to get a coffee frappe and offer some to Graham. Of course, he had never drunk coffee and I wasn't sure if he had ever even tried coffee ice cream. I poured some of the frappe into the plastic "sippy cup" he used for drinking his milk and water and held it up to his lips, not knowing quite what reaction to expect. The ensuing slurping sound could have been heard back at State Beach, as my sunny summer pal drained the cup in one long gulp, punctuated by a tremendous belch that practically rattled the Jeep and resulted in an appreciative cheer from his fellow riders. I refilled his cup and his response was identical, punctuation included.

Graham and I would repeat that indulgence just about as often as we passed Mad Martha's in the years that followed. It became one of those small family traditions that connect generations and symbolize precious time spent with people you love in a special place.

"There is only one happiness in life:
To love and be loved."

—George Sand

I asked a patient of mine some time ago about his family. The Boston bank he worked for had moved him with his wife and children to Luxembourg several years prior to his visit with me. His teenage son and daughter attended an international school there, spoke several languages and had traveled and studied around the world. They had lived among Bedouins, climbed Mount Kilimanjaro and ridden elephants in southeast Asia. One was teaching English for the summer to children in Tanzania and learning Swahili. More importantly, they sounded like wonderfully grounded kids who had been carefully taught about *noblesse oblige* and the satisfaction that comes from assisting others. Their father's pride was wonderful to see. I was impressed by his description of those extraordinary children and struck, of course, by how different our parenting experiences had been. I was happy for my proud patient.

But I was not jealous of him. And I was no less proud of my son than he was of his accomplished children. In very different ways, both of us had enjoyed rich experiences as fathers. It was true that Graham and I would never experience some of the more exotic adventures that my patient described. But, in fact, my son and I had already tackled some very challenging sports that many people are afraid to even try, including skiing and windsurfing. And there was one far less dramatic skill that Graham and I had come very close to mastering. A skill that can be elusive for many families. A skill that is very simple, yet very powerful: *being* together.

Because of health issues and physical challenges, there were times when Graham was limited to staying home with his parents. On those occasions, I began to understand that it was simply being together that made us happy. We didn't have to actually be doing anything in particular. It was fine to be inside during a blizzard. In fact, as it says in the "Christmas Song":

"As long as you love me so, let it snow, let it snow, let it snow!"

I learned to savor the hours we passed in front of a fire in the winter, reading, watching a movie or listening to music. I could feel Graham's nervous system—and my own—calming down on those days. Like his mother, I never failed to tell him how proud we were of his daily effort, his patience and his sense of humor. "You've earned this day of rest, Lad! Today we just chill out!"

On our more challenging days, like those when Graham had a seizure, we developed a habit of listening to *Return to Pooh Corner* by Kenny Loggins and we came to know the whole album by heart. My mom had read *Winnie the Pooh* to me as a child when I wasn't feeling well, and we still had a stuffed Pooh Bear that I had given to my son years ago. Lying side by side on Graham's bed, the music had an uncanny way of helping us to relax and ride out the storm. With my arm around his neck, Graham's eyelids would usually grow heavy as we listened to Kenny's nostalgic words:

> "It's hard to explain how a few precious things
> Seem to follow throughout all our lives
> After all's said and done
> I was watching my son
> Sleeping there with my bear by his side
> I tucked him in, I kissed him
> And as I was going
> I swear that old bear whispered
> 'Boy, welcome home'"

Along a breathtaking bluff in 'Sconset, on the southeastern elbow of the island of Nantucket, sits the historic Sankaty Lighthouse. It was built in 1850 on a ninety-foot cliff above the Atlantic to protect mariners from the dangerous shoals that lurk just off the coastline. When Graham was about two, his Uncle Michael took one of the most beautiful photos ever taken of us near that cliff. Cynthia, Graham and I were on the island in late June, vacationing with Michael and his wife Mary Robb, Cynthia's sister, and their daughter Mariel. In the golden hour before sunset one magnificently clear evening, Michael, Graham and I went for a walk along the bluff. I was carrying Graham on my shoulders when we came to the weathered stone and brick lighthouse.

Michael, a professional videographer with an artist's sense of composition, saw a dramatic metaphor in his mind's eye when Graham and I walked by the structure, outlined in the fading light. He reacted quietly and we didn't know he had taken a picture until he sent us a print weeks later. The image shows a silhouette of Graham and me juxtaposed with the outline of the lighthouse. The Sankaty light's powerful beacon rests on its base of granite and brick as Graham sits on top of my shoulders.

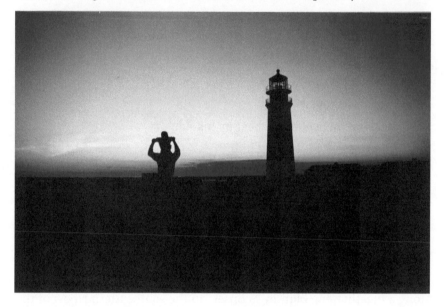

Michael's photo

I wept when I saw it.

Many years after Michael took the picture at the Sankaty Light, Graham and I became acquainted with two astonishing people, a University of Maryland graduate student, Brecken Swartz, and Zhou Lin (Joe-Leen), a Chinese youngster who had been badly burned in rural China at age eleven. Most of Zhou Lin's fingers and toes had been amputated at a small hospital in her remote province during the weeks following an explosion in her home. Incredibly, she was then summarily discharged from that clinic, with no provision for rehabilitation or follow-up care of any kind. In desperation, the youngster's parents, small farmers with few resources, brought the girl to Beijing. They traveled in buses, on the backs of donkeys and, at times, carrying their daughter on their own shoulders, with only a vague plan to beg for help from the Chinese government or even from total strangers.

Brecken Swartz, a vibrant brown-eyed scholar, was engaged in doctoral studies there when she almost literally stumbled upon Zhou Lin among a group of beggars outside a Beijing television studio. In Brecken's words, "My life changed in that moment."

With the blessing of Zhou Lin's family, Brecken brought the girl to Shriner's Hospital in Boston, where she learned to play the dulcimer while Dr. Rob Sheridan performed a lengthy series of surgeries on her. Torturous months later, Zhou Lin was successfully fitted for prosthetic feet.

A hospital administrator suggested that I photograph Brecken and Zhou Lin for a project I was working on at the time about humanism. From the first moment I saw them, I was stunned by the love that so profoundly connected them, two people who had been total strangers not so long before. When I first met Zhou Lin, she was in a wheelchair or using special crutches. A month later, when she and Brecken paid me a visit at my office near Shriner's, Zhou Lin was using a walker, balancing herself on temporary prosthetic feet. The next time I saw her, Zhou Lin walked into my office on her own. No wheelchair, no crutches, no walker.

And she was wearing flip flops.

I wanted Graham to meet Brecken and Zhou Lin, knowing that, like me, he would marvel at their astonishing resilience and the power of love they so beautifully embodied. I knew, too, that they would recognize similar qualities in him. In the late summer, we brought the pair to a beach in Marblehead. It was the first time Zhou Lin had seen the ocean. In the fall, we took them apple picking. Graham and I became friends with those two magical people and, for a short time, they were even our houseguests. Later in the fall, we invited Zhou Lin and Brecken to join a Jabberwocky outing at a Harvard football game. Unsurprisingly, it was a first for a girl from rural China. I offered to get some snacks for the group and asked Zhou Lin what she wanted. "Turnip soup," she replied.

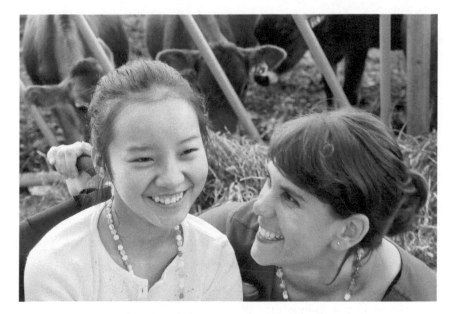

Zhou Lin and Brecken

During one of their visits to our home in Salem, Brecken and Zhou Lin were struck by Michael's memorable photo of Graham and me on Nantucket, which was prominently displayed on a kitchen wall. A few weeks later, they presented us with a coffee table book called *My Dad Fixed the Lighthouse*. The story centers on a boy's excitement when his dad is selected by the Coast Guard to restore the Bakers Island Lighthouse off the coast of Massachusetts. The youngster is ecstatic that he and his family would be spending an entire summer on an island. Brecken and Zhou Lin apparently knew that the Bakers Island Lighthouse was real and, furthermore, that it was conspicuous from the beach where Graham and I kayaked.

Zhou Lin and Brecken inscribed the book with words that mirrored the wonderment and deep fondness we felt for them:

"To a father and son who build
To a father and son who shine light
Helping others find their way in the darkness
We are grateful to be in your lives
And experience a tiny slice of the
Heaven that your strength
And patience and love create
You are a lighthouse
The two of you
Tower and light combined."

There are many fine doctors on the staff of the Harvard Medical School. Some have won Nobel prizes, and others have quietly created ground-breaking programs that have changed lives for the better around the world. Thus it was with absolute astonishment that I received the Harvard Medical School's Humanism in Medicine award one year. The honor was particularly moving because it is awarded by the medical students to one of their mentors. I was nominated by my Primary Care Clerkship student, Jane Unaeze, a dazzling young woman from Nigeria whom I was lucky enough to precept one day a week for a year in my clinic at Massachusetts General Hospital. Some of the other nominees for the award were renowned physicians at Boston teaching hospitals from whom I, myself, had learned medicine. I was stunned to be considered in the same company as those esteemed doctors. I genuinely felt like Ringo Starr of the Beatles who famously asked, "What's a bloke like me doing with these three?"

The award ceremony was at the medical school and, given the once-in-a-lifetime circumstance, I wanted Graham to be there with me. I wanted to pay tribute to my son, to thank him openly for inspiring me every day. And I wanted him to hear me share stories about Camp Jabberwocky and how those experiences had changed me as a physician—and person.

The ceremony was on a weekday and, at the time, Graham was still a residential student at Crotched Mountain. The school graciously offered to transport him from the campus in New Hampshire to Boston in one of their vans for the special occasion, accompanied by a nurse's aide. Rather than try to explain to the van driver how to find the specific location of the event in the maze-like Harvard Medical Area, I suggested that the van simply meet me at the main entrance to Children's Hospital that is adjacent to the campus. I took a cab across Boston from my office at MGH, still attired in a white doctor's jacket from my morning clinic and waited in front of the world-renowned hospital for children.

Right on time, the Crotched Mountain minivan pulled up at the hospital entrance and the aide pushed Graham down a metal ramp in his wheelchair. I was thrilled to see my son, who looked like a Ralph Lauren model in a special outfit Lisa had chosen for him, featuring his blue blazer. I was not consciously thinking about it at the time, but, subliminally, some part of me was probably aware of how close Graham had come to dying there at Children's Hospital just a few years earlier. By contrast, on the day of the medical school ceremony, emerging from the Crotched Mountain van, Graham was the embodiment of robust health. When we made eye contact, my whole being filled with joy.

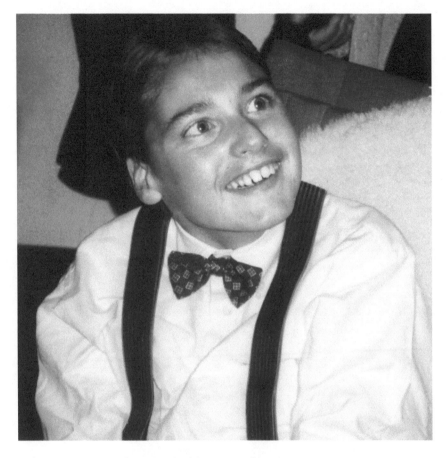

Dressed for a special occasion

Still wearing my white jacket, I greeted Graham in front of the hospital with a barrage of hugs and kisses even more extravagant than those he normally tolerated so patiently from Cynthia and me. It happened at that moment that an elderly, snow-haired matron was passing us in a walker with a companion holding her by the arm. As they shuffled by, I heard the older lady whisper to her friend, "Gracious … the doctors at this hospital are awfully affectionate with their patients!"

7

HEROES AMONG US

A special thrill for Graham and me during his Crotched Mountain years was visiting our friends, the Reids, in Fitzwilliam, New Hampshire, at the pastoral farm that had been in their family since 1930. Dr. David Reid, well into his eighties by then, had been my family doctor growing up and the father of four childhood friends in the Boston suburb of Weston, Massachusetts. Later, he encouraged me when I was considering medical school and became my first mentor. Dave was a role model for me as a doctor and a father. He and his wife, Jean, spent summers in Fitzwilliam, often joined by Dave's sons, David, Robby and Billy, his daughter Betsy and assorted spouses, grandchildren, pets and friends. The old farmhouse was typically filled with the uninhibited laughter and general cacophony of a big, loving family. Dave had steady blue eyes, wispy remnants of white hair and a dry sense of humor.

The farm at Fitzwilliam was only about forty minutes from Crotched Mountain. Graham and I would make a date to come over for lunch once or twice during the summer, enjoying visits with our old friends in a setting straight out of Robert Frost's New England—a big barn, ancient stone walls and thick stands of birches and fir trees. On our visits to the farm, Dave and his whole family embraced Graham without hesitation and made us feel absolutely welcome in their home. There was a hammock behind the farmhouse that Graham particularly enjoyed. Dave's sons would carefully carry Graham from his wheelchair onto the hammock and we would sit around it, with Graham in the middle of the group. It was wonderful to reminisce about the life we had shared in Weston in an earlier time when Dave made house calls after dinner in a rusty station wagon, accompanied by his golden retriever, Rory.

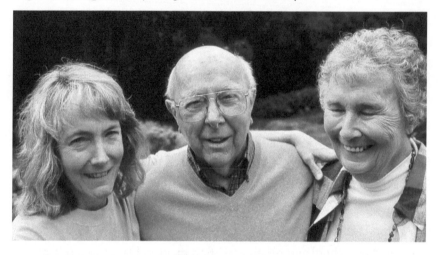

Dave with daughter Betsy and wife Jean

Dave passed away at ninety, and Graham and I were part of a large congregation in the Fitzwilliam Community Church that celebrated his life. At the memorial service, we learned that his favorite poem had been Frost's "Stopping by Woods on a Snowy Evening." Fitzwilliam could have been the bucolic setting for that famous poem, and Dave, who made some evening house calls even after turning eighty, might well have been the narrator who observed:

> "The woods are lovely dark and deep.
> But I have promises to keep,

And miles to go before I sleep,
And miles to go before I sleep."

Only at Dave's memorial service did I learn that he had come ashore as a newly minted physician among the first wave of allied troops at Normandy in the hours following the D-Day invasion, and that he had managed a field hospital on Utah Beach. Keeping such information to himself was typical of his humility. Dave quietly did what was honorable, like others among that "Greatest Generation" which, as Tom Brokaw wrote, "made no demands of homage from those who followed and prospered because of its sacrifices."

On our visits to Fitzwilliam, Dave was always curious about Graham's progress and our adventures together. Visiting with a warm and attentive friend who had known me since I was a little boy—for half a century—was a rare pleasure. Feeling Dave's respect and encouragement was poignant. He was not one to offer praise carelessly and, when he spoke, his words were from the heart. After one of our visits to the farm, I received a note written in my old friend's nearly illegible scribble, the product of some sixty years as a busy doctor. I knew that writing cards at that stage of his life was probably something he didn't do often. It simply said, "Hi Steve, It was nice to see you and Graham again. It is easy to see that he knows how much you love him. You should both be proud. Love to you both, Dave."

Graham and I were looking for an opportunity to test ourselves and have some fun at the same time. We wanted to do something athletic, but, ideally, something that would also make us feel good spiritually. We were aware of the hugely successful annual bicycle event called the Pan Mass Challenge that raises money for the Jimmy Fund, the charity that supports pioneering research and patient care at the Dana Farber Cancer Institute in Boston. In the past, we had enjoyed riding a special tandem bicycle that was owned by our friend Jonathan Traquina, a Jabberwocky camper who lived near Boston. We were sure that Jonathan would lend us his bike. But, were we up to the demands of the PMC?

If we did it, we could dedicate our ride to the memory of our special friend from Camp Jabberwocky, Virginia Hackney, who had succumbed to pancreatic cancer.

We checked out the PMC website together. There were shorter options besides the 200-mile two-day ride from Sturbridge in central Massachusetts out to the tip of Cape Cod in Provincetown. One option that looked good to us was a one-day loop that started and ended in the Boston suburb of Wellesley and was considerably shorter. Since we would be riding a fairly heavy bike with only three gears, the Wellesley option seemed the better part of valor. We would need Cynthia's help for logistical and moral support along the way, not to mention food and drinks. She was game and volunteered to provision and drive our "support car."

Graham and I considered carefully whether this was something we could do. It would require training and commitment. For one thing, there was a significant fundraising responsibility, which meant writing letters and keeping track of donations. For another, we would need to be out on the road on the day of the event for at least four hours. The weather in August in New England was hard to predict. It might be sweltering with oppressive humidity or raining torrentially.

I explained all this in detail, making sure Graham understood what we were getting into. He never hesitated. He looked right at me, and his whole body seemed to contract into a big grin, punctuated by a loud vocalization that simply said, "Dad, we're doing it!"

And we did. With abundant help from Cynthia, on what turned out to be a perfect summer day, we rode nearly forty miles together. Graham, who had woken up at three in the morning and nearly leaped out of bed with excitement, looked straight ahead during the event, sitting confidently in front of me while I pumped the pedals. When I felt depleted on some of the longer uphill climbs, I found strength in the words of Dick Hoyt, the father who has pushed his disabled son Rick in a racing wheelchair in scores of marathons and other demanding events: "Rick is the real athlete. I am only lending him some muscle power."

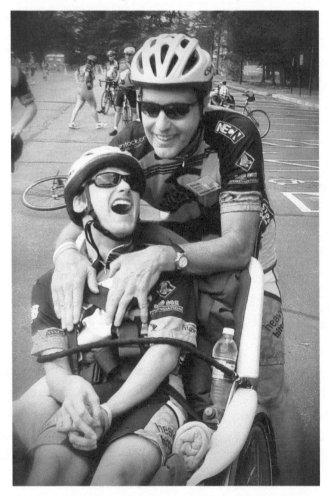

Before the Pan Mass Challenge

I felt the same way on that halcyon summer day. It was Graham who broke the wind for us, looking strong and cool in his sleek sunglasses and the wildly colorful racing uniform that all the PMC riders wore that day. Although I couldn't see his face, I could feel the poise of the athlete in front of me. I rode in Graham's slipstream on that special day. Later, I examined the beautiful photos that Cynthia took of us during our ride, and I was struck by the expression in Graham's intense hazel eyes. I saw a determination to achieve a kind of personal best. But there was something else. Graham knew that the PMC was more than a bike ride. He knew that he was part of an effort to help people facing adversity. He was happy and proud.

"In all this time we traveled together something happened.
Something I'll have to think about for a long time."
—Ernesto Guevera, *The Motorcycle Diaries*

Graham and I had a favorite movie, *The Motorcycle Diaries,* the story of Ernesto ("Che") Guevara, a twenty-three-year-old medical student from Buenos Aires, and his friend, Alberto Granado, on their epic journey around South America on an aging, cantankerous Norton 500 motorcycle. The story begins as a youthful "road trip," but subtly evolves into something more profound—the young men's growing awareness of the vast disparity between the privileged and the underclasses on their continent. Ernesto's epiphany is symbolized in a poignant scene in which he makes a dangerous swim across the Amazon River to the leper colony of San Pablo, Peru. There, he physically and metaphorically bonds with the patients, pariahs who normally have no contact with the rest of society. The swim bridges the gulf between the healthy and the unhealthy, the haves and have-nots and represents the turning point in Che's life.

Graham and I watched the movie together several times, lying side-by-side on his bed. On car trips, we listened to the beautiful soundtrack, poignant instrumental music that somehow seemed mournful and hopeful at the same time. I began to call Graham "Ernesto" or "Fuser" (Few-say), Alberto's pet name for his best friend. Like Ernesto, Graham was handsome, charismatic and scrupulously honest. He was literally incapable of being disingenuous. When Graham gave you a smile, it was real. And, like the young Che, Graham interacted in an open-hearted way with the people he met, regardless of their social status.

The adapted three-speed tandem bicycle that Graham and I rode in the PMC was a far cry from Ernesto and Alberto's Norton 500, but, nonetheless, we identified with them. When I looked at Graham, I *saw* Ernesto, because he represented people who are normally invisible in our world. Like Ernesto and Alberto, Graham and I were transformed by our journey, both the PMC bike ride itself and our larger odyssey through life dealing with a profound disability. At Camp Jabberwocky and Crotched Mountain, we met people with "handicaps" who stunned us with their courage and resilience. We saw how much fun they had and how readily they were able to live in the present. We saw them try difficult activities without self-consciousness. We saw people of different abilities assisting one another and testing limits. As Ernesto says in his diary, "This isn't a tale of heroic feats. It's about two lives running parallel for a while, with common aspirations and similar dreams."

Graham changed me. I am no longer the same man that I was before. In all the time we traveled together, something happened—something I will have to think about for a long time.

Watching the enthusiastic throng along the route of the Pan Mass Challenge, I was reminded of the huge, appreciative crowds that greet Camp

Jabberwocky every summer at the Fourth of July Parade in Edgartown. The spectacular midsummer event has been a tradition on the island for decades, and the Jabberwocky campers and counselors who "march" in it invariably receive the loudest reception from the massive gathering. Passionate cheering swells as the campers, many in wheelchairs, navigate the four-mile route past nineteenth-century whaling captain's houses, through one of the most picturesque coastal villages in the world.

Against the breathtaking backdrop of Edgartown's harbor and gray-shingled cottages surrounded by rose gardens and privet hedges, Camp Jabberwocky always seems to take center stage. Dressed in outrageous costumes that resonate with a playful theme and riding in ingenious "floats," typically created in the wee hours of that very morning by counselors running on adrenaline, Camp Jabberwocky shines with all its magic on America's birthday.

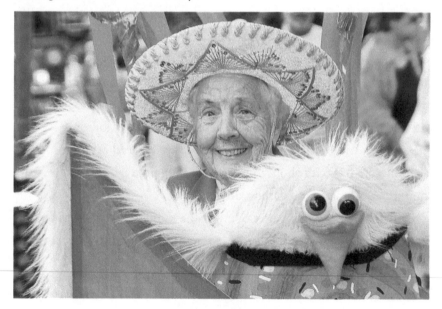

Hellcat at the parade

When Graham was introduced to Camp, thanks to Cynthia's friend Lisa Dold, a longtime counselor, we quickly learned that the parade was the highlight of the July camp session, the ultimate opportunity for them to strut their stuff. In the years that followed, I took hundreds of photos of the campers and counselors dressed up as characters from movies like *Jaws* and *Pirates of the Caribbean* and put them into slide shows that we laughed at later during "Studio Night," Camp's irreverent weekly variety show.

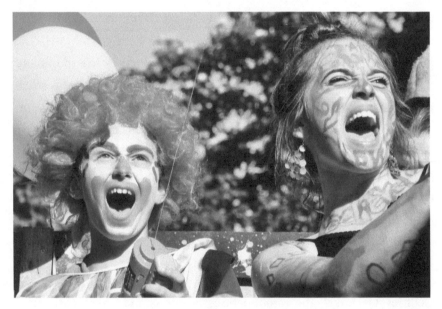

Shawn and Adrian squirt the crowd

One year, however, I decided to turn my camera around and focus on the spectators who lined the parade route. I wanted to see if I could capture the emotion that seemed to impassion the people watching Camp. I began by zooming in on the crowd from a flat-bed truck in front of the Camp procession. Then I dropped back and took shots from various angles while walking among the campers. The faces in the resulting photos were diverse, including aristocratic Brahmins in ascots, towheaded children in Ralph Lauren polos and local fishermen in funky T-shirts. Yet, nearly uniformly, the spectators were embracing Camp. In some places, the crowd was ten deep. Boisterous groups hoisting adult beverages cheered madly from balconies and rooftops. The energy reminded me of the full-throated throngs in Boston that cheer the appearance of the first runners and wheelchair athletes along the Boston Marathon route on Patriots' Day.

Jabberwocky has enriched the Vineyard with its unconventional presence for almost seven decades, and the island community has, in turn, supported Camp in many generous ways. It is a nice symbiosis. The people who line the parade route are clearly touched by the spunk and resilience of the campers. While they come to applaud, they also relish the opportunity to laugh with the campers, to absorb and celebrate Jabberwocky's knack for seizing the day and having fun.

Over the years, I felt goosebumps watching thousands of onlookers unabashedly cheering for Graham as he was pushed along the parade route, costumed as a Willy Wonka elevator, a Wimbledon tennis champion, a Pirate of the Caribbean, a punk rocker—and an octopus.

Geoffrey Garfinkel, the rambunctious leader of the Therapeutic Recreation Department at Crotched Mountain, taught Graham and me to ski together. It turned out to be a monumental gift. Skiing was both a thrilling sport and an opportunity to experience the soulfulness of wintertime in New England. Being able to actually enjoy winter high in the White Mountains was making lemonade out of lemons during the dreary months when many locals were griping about the cold and feeling trapped indoors.

At Crotched Mountain, as well as Mount Sunapee and Wachusett Mountain, Geoff showed me how to tether Graham with nylon straps attached to a "sit ski," an adaptive device with a bucket seat mounted on a pair of short skis. In this adaptive version of skiing, the companion skier (the "tetherer") snowplows behind the disabled skier in the seat and helps steer and control speed with the straps. With a little practice, the two tandem skiers can turn or skid to a stop—preferably when they want to! Graham and I produced some impressive bloopers and "yard sales" while learning this new skill. In ski parlance, a yard sale occurs when a skier falls clumsily and slides helter-skelter downhill, leaving mittens, goggles, skis and ski poles behind in an embarrassing trail of debris. Graham gave me a sardonic grin the first time he saw me upside down in the snow, missing a ski, while he had somehow remained upright.

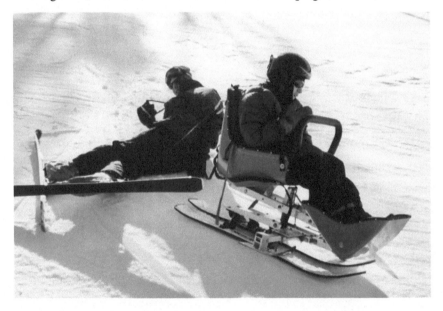

A minor yard sale

I had loved skiing ever since college, but until Geoff and his colleague, Becca Krest, showed us the world of adaptive skiing, it had never occurred to me that Graham and I might be able to enjoy the demanding sport together. Dancing down powdery, tree-lined alpine trails, with Graham once again in the lead, we discovered a fresh sense of freedom. High in the White Mountains on a sun-splashed January day, during a time of year so often hostile in our part of the world, winter revealed its glory to the two of us. As we descended a trail at Crotched Mountain called Big Dipper, I thrilled at the sight of my son's helmeted head bobbing in front of me and realized that I was experiencing something very close to euphoria. If Geoff had given me the Hope Diamond and the deed to a gold mine, I would not have been as ecstatic as I was in those moments.

As the mountain steepened just a little, we picked up speed and found a steady rhythm. At the bottom of the trail, I had to blink away some warm drops of moisture that had fogged the inside of my goggles before sharing an exuberant bear hug with my son.

Ernie Dilisio was a gaunt but endearing rapscallion who repaired golf clubs in a small shop at his modest home in Swampscott, a town near us. He was in poor health, and everyone who cared about him gave him grief about his chain smoking. When Ernie opened his front door, a dense cloud of smoke usually gushed out, delivering a noxious plume of tobacco toxins into the nostrils of his customers. I learned to hold my breath after knocking on that door. Ernie was absent-minded and some-times had several cigarettes burning at the same time in different parts of the dim apartment. It was not unusual to find a few Marlboros smolder-ing on the carpet next to the sofa where he napped. The ambiance of the place fit my mental image of an opium den.

Ernie had a litany of insecurities and quirks, but his heart was even bigger than the cloud of smoke that filled his home. A golfer I knew had told me about Ernie, and one day I went over to meet him and have new grips put on my clubs. Graham was in the passenger seat of the car, and Ernie wobbled down a rickety set of steps to greet him. Something about meeting Graham visibly affected Ernie. I spotted tears glistening in his eyes as he held precariously onto the railing by his front steps and watched us pull away.

When I knocked on the door of Ernie's place a week later to collect my re-gripped golf clubs, he emerged like a ghost materializing out of a wall of fog and handed me a gift, the first of many he would give us. It was a hand-crafted golf club, cut down to Graham's size and adapted so that it could be swung, with assistance, from a wheelchair. Ernie had worked on it for many hours that week.

About a month later, I was spending a fall weekend at Crotched Mountain with Graham. As usual, Lisa was helping us, and we decided to try out Graham's new club at a local golf course. The greenskeeper there kindly allowed us to take Graham's wheelchair out on a vacant fairway and we whacked some balls around, resulting in a series of errant shots known to golfers as "worm burners" and "foozles." But it was a sunny autumn after-noon in New England, and simply being out in the brisk mountain air with Graham and his trusty friend was delightful. We didn't care much about where the balls ended up.

When most of the balls had, in fact, ended up in the woods, we decided we had played enough golf for one day and headed for what all golfers know as the "nineteenth hole." We had brought Graham's supper with us, and the kitchen in the little tavern connected to the clubhouse gladly warmed it for us while Lisa and I ordered something from the menu. It happened that afternoon that the restaurant was crowded with golfers watching the Little League World Series on big-screen televisions. There was a table available in the back of the pub and we took it, a little tired but pleased to have added a new sport to our repertoire.

From our location, the nearest TV was blocked by a boisterous group at a crowded table right in from of us. From their loud merriment, it was clear that those sportsmen had punctuated their round of golf with a few libations. I sensed that they were mildly uncomfortable with us in their midst, probably not being used to having a youngster in a wheelchair with cerebral palsy at their favorite watering hole. But a moment later, one of them, a portly fellow with a Friar Tuck haircut, came over and asked if they were blocking Graham's view of the Little League World Series. I told him not to worry about it, but, before we could protest, the entire gang of seven or eight golfing pals had lifted up their table, crammed with precariously oscillating plates and glasses, and put it down some five feet to the side, so that Graham could have a clear view of the game.

It seemed to me that, for the next hour or so, those guys kept making up excuses to drop by our table and ask if Graham needed anything. One lanky fellow with a walrus mustache asked if Graham enjoyed chocolate cake. About a minute later, our waitress placed a huge piece of German chocolate cake in front of Graham, compliments of our new friends.

As Thanksgiving approached, Graham and I planned a trip to see my cousins in the rustic town of Sherman, Connecticut. Veteran travelers between Boston and New York who crave a mouthwatering corned beef sandwich know that you exit Interstate 84 in the town of Vernon, near Hartford, and stop at the venerable restaurant called Rein's New York Deli. I pushed Graham into the crammed restaurant lobby, where we were greeted by Monica AuClair, one of the establishment's managers. This total stranger, a beaming, lithe young woman, walked up to Graham's wheelchair in the middle of the hectic lunch hour, gazed right at him and said, "Who is this incredibly handsome young man who has graced us with his presence on this beautiful day?"

Over the years, we went out of our way to stop at Rein's on our occasional trips to Connecticut, always hoping that our radiant friend was still there. She always was, and she never failed to greet Graham with the same effusive enthusiasm. Even when the deli was chaotically busy, Monica sat down to visit with us as if we were the only people in the room. Whenever we saw Monica, I thought about kindness. From years of watching strangers respond to Graham, including Ernie Dilisio and the golfers at Crotched Mountain, I had become convinced that a major-ity of people are inherently warm-hearted. In the bedlam of Rein's New York Deli in Vernon, Connecticut, Monica AuClair was the unaffected embodiment of what the Dalai Lama calls his "simple religion":

"Be kind whenever possible. It is always possible."

One Halloween, the singularly boisterous holiday in the town of Salem where I live, Graham and I dressed up as Batman and Robin. The Batman suit was the larger of the two, so I wore that, and Graham wore the Robin costume. Subliminally at first, I began to remember a conversation that had taken place several years earlier in my office with a patient who worked at a comic book store in Boston. He had told me that avid fans of the "Dynamic Duo" do not consider Robin a secondary superhero lan-guishing in the shadow of Batman. Instead, Robin is viewed by some as the real moral compass of the pair.

While I had given Graham the Robin outfit for the simple reason that it was the smaller of the two, I began to think more carefully about the choice. My patient's notion that Robin was the real conscience of the two-some resonated with a conviction that had been growing in me: Graham had a pureness of heart that was vanishingly rare in our world. Long before we picked out costumes for Halloween that year, I had started to believe that—if my son and I were any kind of dynamic duo—I was the sidekick. Like a comic book crusader, Graham's moral code was impeccable. He had never hurt a single person in his life. He had never told a lie. He had never failed a friend.

It seemed to me that Cynthia and I were moving into a more rewarding phase of our lives on the coattails of our son. Because she and I could speak and walk, it appeared to outside observers that we were in charge. But we had both begun to feel that we were here to lend our voices and muscle power to a person whose goodness far exceeded our own. Others who knew Graham and assisted him were feeling that they, too, were part of a supporting cast. Foremost among them was Lisa, his truest friend and helper, who was pushing Graham's wheelchair that Halloween, a pirate in red capri pants with flowing blond curls. In Lisa's heart, Graham had been a model of grace and the star of our show for a long time.

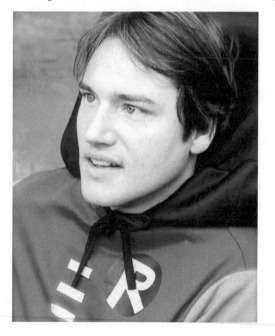

Robin

As the flaxen-haired pirate pushed Robin in his black cape and green tights through the raucous crowd in Salem that day, I sensed that I was

watching art imitating life. The young man dressed as a comic book crusader was, in fact, a real-life superhero.

Graham's grandmother, my mom, died peacefully in hospice care during
the Christmas season of 2005 at the age of eighty-one. She passed away
with the dignity that so characterized her life. She was ready to let go of
this life and was unafraid. Mom's gradual decline played out over a period
of weeks at a hospice house near my brother's home. Will and I were with
her much of the time, along with Will's wife, Linda, but, after a while, we
took turns going to work and attending to our more mundane responsibilities. One evening I went to see Mom at the facility as the end was
clearly getting closer. She had essentially stopped eating and was on mor-
phine. I wanted to take her a treat of some kind, and the only appealing
thing that I could find in my poorly-provisioned kitchen was a perfectly
ripe Bartlett pear.

At her bedside, I sliced it into thin strips, the width of a wafer, and
tentatively placed one on her tongue, acutely aware of the role reversal we
were playing out. How many times had she fed Will and me as infants?
How much of her entire life, in fact, had been invested in providing for
us? The sweet flavor of the pear and the moisture in her dry mouth must
have been pleasing. The muscles over her high cheekbones rose just per-
ceptibly and, for the last time, I saw a hint of the beautiful smile that had
once illuminated the covers of magazines during her career as a fashion
model in New York City.

I went to work the next day struggling to distract myself from the
epochal event about to happen. When I came home, I put on some
Christmas music and had a snack while preparing for the short ride to
the hospice center. The phone rang, however, and Will told me that Mom
was gone. She had fallen asleep peacefully and simply stopped breathing.

I put the phone down and sat quietly, letting the reality of his words sink in. A subliminal part of me became aware of the Christmas carol that was playing in my living room. Its unmistakable melody evoked memories of the Christmas seasons of my life and the people I have loved across the generations of my family.

Emerging from my reverie, I became consciously aware of the song that was playing. Mom had played it herself on the piano for us as children on Christmas Eve. I settled back into the couch, allowing the comforting words of its refrain to wash over me: "Sleep in Heavenly Peace. Sleep in Heavenly Peace."

Several days later, I opened a Christmas package from Graham and Donna Chadwick, his phenomenal music therapist at Crotched Mountain. I knew that it would contain a cassette of their work together that semester, a gift that I anticipated and treasured every year during the holiday season. I had been saving it for about a week, waiting to open it at just the right moment. I found an old boom box and plugged in the cassette. First, Donna introduced their project for that semester, *Christmas Music,* and described Graham's hard work on it. Graham's assignment had been to use his voice as much as he could while Donna sang and, also, to help record the songs. Donna had been teaching Graham to coordinate one of his hands to hit a big button she had attached to a tray in the front of his wheelchair, a task that was difficult for him. When pressed, the button started and stopped a recording.

During Donna's introduction, I heard Graham's voice in the background, laughing. He had successfully hit the button that started the recording. I then heard Donna's lovely voice singing:

"Silent night, holy night
All is calm, all is bright
'Round yon virgin Mother and Child
Holy infant so tender and mild
Sleep in heavenly peace
Sleep in heavenly peace."

Donna then wished me a Merry Christmas, on behalf of Graham, and asked him to hit the button to stop the recording. I heard them both giggle for a moment, followed by a loud thump and, then—silence.

"Oh how we will miss our frequent encounters
with Graham and Cynthia during their walk through
the neighborhood. His smiling greetings were unsurpassed.
There is now a hole in our hearts."
—Mary and Gary Ritter

Cynthia took Graham on vigorous walks around Marblehead Neck whenever he was home on weekends and vacations. They ventured forth in all seasons, even on blustery days in the fall and winter when the hardiest locals were curled up by a wood fire. Graham loved the unpredictable and sometimes extreme New England weather. He was not afraid of getting wet, and he did not mind the wind gusting in his face as he and his mom crossed the open causeway en route to their hilly loop around Marblehead Neck with its spectacular ocean vistas.

Graham would look straight ahead, bundled up according to the season in his blue canvas jogger with its big wheels, enjoying the sensation of speed and the ever-changing elements of nature in New England. In rain or snow, Graham would stick out his tongue to get a taste of the precipitation tickling his face. Cynthia, about the same size as her son, but with a gymnast's athleticism, could push Graham as fast as most joggers run on their own and sing to him at the same time. In the dead of winter, only a handful of the most rugged lobstermen remained at work at moorings in the harbor. Cynthia recognized three sturdy boats that always seemed to be on the water braving the elements with Graham and her in what felt like a curious kind of solidarity. One was white, one red, and one turquoise.

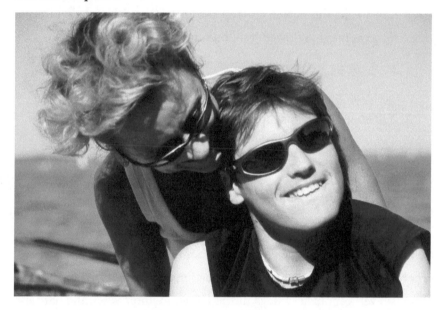

Bud, have I told you today how much I love you?

Graham and his mom had a favorite place on the route that they referred to as their "outdoor cafe" where they would stop for Cynthia to give Graham a drink and admire the ocean views. They found another special spot halfway around the Neck where birds were always singing. On the homeward leg of the outings, Cynthia would make sure that her boy was sitting in a good position before crossing the causeway where they could see the Boston skyline to the south and Marblehead harbor to the north. Along that stretch, they would periodically slow down and listen to the sea lashing the reinforced retaining walls of the causeway. Cynthia had an impression that the rhythmic ebb and flow of waves on the gravel beach facing the Atlantic sounded like applause swelling and receding in a theater.

On those trips around Marblehead Neck, Graham would frequently be greeted by his "fans," as Cynthia called them. Neighbors of different backgrounds would run with them for a while or shout greetings to this "Prince of Marblehead" and his mom. Bikes would stop and people would emerge from homes as if the Pied Piper himself were passing. And about every fifteen minutes, Cynthia would stop for a moment, bend over and repeat the same question to her handsome companion:

"Bud, have I told you today how much I love you?"

On a balmy late August weekend, Graham and I had some father and son time scheduled and Cynthia had a rare weekend free. She decided to get out of town and take her vintage Volvo sports coupe on a run. She always felt liberated on the road in her clay blue "baby," the classic sports car driven by Roger Moore in the 1960s television spy series *The Saint*. She decided upon Woodstock, Vermont, and called Jim, an old friend, whose family had a home there, to get his recommendation for lodging. He told her the only lodging she would need was his family house, and Cynthia and her clay blue baby were on the road.

Three hours later, she crossed a covered wooden bridge and found the address. Before her was a stately home with a portico nestled at the base of Mount Tom, formally a small ski area. Behind the house, at the edge of a dense woodland, were an ancient barn and gazebo. Cynthia had a premonition that something magical might be in store for her in that picturesque destination at the edge of the Green Mountains. Jim had told her that she could climb Mount Tom directly from the back of the property, and she promptly dropped her bag and headed up, scrambling along a wooded path that wound its way to the 1,250-foot summit of the gentle mountain. Periodically, Cynthia would turn and watch Jim's home receding further into what increasingly resembled one of those idyllic miniature villages in a model train layout.

In less than a half-hour, she reached the summit and admired the rustic hamlet of Woodstock nestled in its valley. On the mountaintop, Cynthia stumbled upon the enormous wrought iron Christmas star that is illuminated during the holiday season and is visible for miles down the Connecticut River Valley. After a brief rest on the summit, Cynthia spotted a wide, cleared path and decided to follow it down. As she inhaled the woodsy fragrance of spruce and fir trees, she noted the trail's gentle pitch and an idea came to her—this might be the perfect place for Graham to add hiking to his growing resume of adventures.

When she got home, she told Graham that she was making plans for them to travel to Woodstock and that, if he was game, they would be hiking to the top of Mount Tom. She talked it up for two weeks, made reservations at the Woodstock Inn, cooked and froze a couple of Graham's favorite meals and tuned up the big canvas jogger that she would be using to push her son up the trail. In his unique fashion, Graham showed his mother that he was psyched for the adventure. On the appointed day, after checking in at the historic Woodstock Inn, Cynthia rolled Graham excitedly across the town green. After a few false starts, they found the Mount Tom path and started off. Both were in high spirits on an invigorating September day.

As Cynthia hit the first incline, however, she realized that she was in for a much more arduous outing than she had expected. She hadn't calculated the effort required to push more than her own weight up a very steep hill over rocky terrain. Looking at Graham, she murmured, "Bud, this is really hard, and I'm not quite sure I can do it." In response, the young man in the jogger turned his head in a movement Cynthia had never seen him make and looked at her as if to say, "Are you kidding? You've talked this up for weeks now, so let's get going!"

Whenever Cynthia would groan, even a little, her companion seemed to turn his head with a benevolent gaze that said, "You can do it, I know you can." Although it seemed at times beyond her strength, Cynthia persevered, periodically rewarded by those encouraging glances from her boy. At the summit, with spectacular vistas of Vermont farms and woodlands extending in every direction, they stopped near the Christmas Star and soaked in the magnificent scene in a moment of shared triumph.

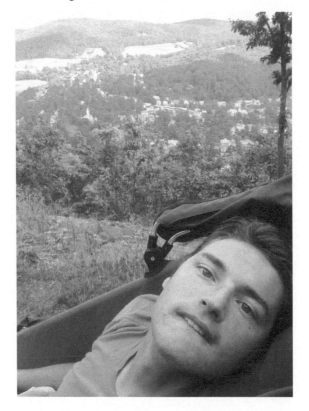

On the summit of Mount Tom

8

SPRING BREAK

Even if you love snow, winter in New England can get depressing. There are lengthy stretches of time when it's dim, dreary... and cold. For people who require a wheelchair, the additional challenges of ice, slush and biting wind can become downright demoralizing. With that in mind, when he was fourteen or fifteen years old, I suggested to Graham that we treat ourselves to an annual April getaway to a tropical destination, our version of "spring break." It would be our prize for surviving the long, dark winter. In addition, it would serve as a reward for a couple of Graham's special friends and helpers who took care of him during the week at Crotched Mountain. We were pretty sure they would be happy to join us.

We picked Nassau as our destination on the first of those tropical holidays. Graham and I cleared customs there with three excited helpers, including his primary one-to-one aides at school, Lisa and Angela and Angela's husband, Adam. Emerging from the terminal, we stopped and inhaled the fragrance of jasmine and luxuriated in the warmth of the sun on our faces for the first time in many months. On our short ride to the resort, it was almost shocking to see *color.* Just a few hours removed from the endless gray of New England in winter, the vivid green crowns of citrus trees and the vibrant yellow and pink hibiscus blossoms were dazzling.

We arrived at our hotel early enough to throw our bags in our rooms and head for the beach in the afternoon. It was a flawless Bahamian day with a gentle breeze. The shoreline wasn't crowded, and the turquoise water beckoned. As I scanned the wide beach, I realized that it would be a struggle to push Graham's big canvas jogger through the unusually soft white sand. At that same moment, I vaguely noticed a muscle-bound man about twenty feet away from us. His skin was a deep shade of brown. I noted an abundance of tattoos and gold chains. He had huge biceps and bulging pectoral muscles and wore a baseball cap backward on his head.

As boys, our mother liked to read the Rudyard Kipling poem, "If," to my brother and me, and I had hung her calligraphed version of it on Graham's wall at Crotched Mountain. Mom believed in treating "paupers and kings" just the same and wanted us to know from an early age that stereotyping people is wrong. I've tried to follow her example over the years and pride myself on judging people on their own merits. But on that glorious afternoon in Nassau, an unkind thought passed involuntarily through my mind—*Whoa…if funky dudes like him are staying here, what kind of a resort have I gotten us into?*

Amazingly, at the exact moment that the disparaging thought passed through my mind, the man started walking directly toward us. Had he read my mind? And, if so, was he about to alter my face? Thankfully, he hadn't read my mind. Nor did he have any intention of hurting anyone. The powerful stranger walked right up to Graham, smiled down at him and turned to me with a grin from ear to ear.

"Hey guys, my name is Benny. I'm not the brightest guy in the world, but I'm strong as an ox. If I could assist you with this special young man in any way while you're here, it would be my honor to do so. Just say the word."

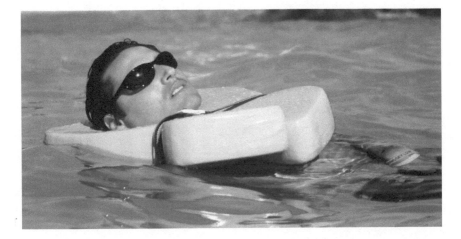

Nassau

And Benny wasn't grandstanding. Whenever he saw us approaching the beach, he would run up, grab Graham and his jogger like a toy and carry them over to our spot on the shoreline. Benny must have discreetly kept an eye on us throughout the day, too, because he seemed to routinely reappear at the exact moment when Graham needed a lift back across the sand.

For our tropical trips, Graham and his team needed theme music. The pop-reggae of UB40 became our choice as the soundtrack for our vacations, and we played and replayed their music in hotel rooms and on the beaches of the Virgin Islands, the Bahamas, Florida and Bermuda. For me, there was nothing more exquisite than seeing a smile on Graham's face after a day at the beach as we said goodnight in a hotel room overlooking the Caribbean, a warm breeze filling our room with tropical scents and UB40 playing in the background. The British group's cover of the old Sonny and Cher hit "I Got You Babe" especially resonated with us:

"So put your little hand in mine
There ain't no hill or mountain we can't climb
I got you to hold my hand
I got you to understand
I got you to walk with me
I got you to talk with me
I got you to kiss good night
I got you to hold me tight
I got you and won't let go
I got you to love me so
I got you babe."

As hokey and simplistic as they sound, Sonny Bono's lyrics "spoke" to us. We already knew a little something about climbing mountains. Graham had reached mountaintops with his mom and dad—in three states. Holding hands, reading each other's moods, walking and talking— those were old habits now that brought us joy every day. As for having someone "to kiss good night," well—with apologies to Graham—we had probably carried that one a bit far over the years. And, holding him any tighter would not have been possible, even with Krazy Glue.

Of course, the last lines of the song summed it all up—we had each other to love.

And, with due respect to the French writer George Sand, we had figured out for ourselves a long time ago that having *that* was "the one true happiness in life."

For one of our spring break adventures, Graham and I flew with Lisa to Vero Beach on the east coast of Florida. We spent a tranquil week there with my cousin, Sandy, as guests in the relaxing home of my brother,

Clint, and his wife Cary, on the breezy barrier beach between the Atlantic Ocean and the Indian River. We rented a red Sebring convertible and savored the warm air on our way out to dinner at night with the top down. We watched a spring training ballgame between the Cardinals and Dodgers from a special section. Minor league players who seemed impossibly young and strong sat just a few feet away from us, and a handful went out of their way to visit with Graham in his wheelchair.

It was a restful vacation, mostly spent lounging around the pool. Graham and I were overjoyed to be away from the bone-chilling world we had left behind. After a week, we packed reluctantly for the trip home. On the flight to Boston, we were sitting in the front row of the plane when my worst fear materialized. Without warning, Graham had a grand mal seizure, accompanied by violent muscle contractions. In seconds he was unconscious, and his face turned an ashen color. I had a medicine that could be given as an injection for seizures that last longer than five minutes and, thankfully, I did not have to use it. After an unnerving few minutes, the seizure stopped on its own.

Following those attacks, Graham typically had what neurologists call "motor restlessness." His muscles would tense and twitch, and he would struggle mightily with his body. He was understandably frightened and upset by the betrayal of his own nervous system. Graham was so physically strong that, after a seizure, it was hard to keep him in a seated position. His back and neck muscles would arch backward involuntarily. During the last hour of the flight, it took all of my physical and mental strength just to keep Graham in his seat while trying everything in my repertoire to comfort him.

It was a tense situation, with nearby passengers and the flight attendants anxiously watching us. I worried that an airline regulation might mandate that the pilot land at the nearest airport. Graham had come out of the seizure, and the last thing I wanted then was to be stranded somewhere in Georgia or South Carolina. But the flight crew remained calm and allowed me to manage the crisis with Lisa's assistance. We made it back to Boston safely, but thoroughly exhausted. I had used all of my reserves of emotional strength to manage the situation.

Graham's mom met us in the baggage area, and I got on an elevator to take our cumbersome collection of luggage and paraphernalia up to the parking level. I recognized a man and two small children in the elevator who had been on our flight. They had been seated a couple of rows behind us and, apparently, had witnessed our entire struggle. At that moment, I was completely spent and aware that I was fighting back tears of relief and exhaustion. My feelings were in turmoil. On one hand, there was anguish that Graham had to suffer through those horrific episodes. On the other was an acute sense of deliverance that we had made it home safely.

Yet, even in those moments of abject weariness, I was overwhelmed by something else—the awareness of how much I could love someone. Caring for this boy, even under the most difficult of circumstances, was a profound privilege and a blessing. I became aware that the young father in the elevator was looking closely at me. Quietly and slowly, with tears welling in his eyes, he said, "Your son—he's a lucky boy." As I pushed the luggage cart out of the elevator, I accepted his handshake and thanked him, knowing that a stranger had just given me the most meaningful compliment I would receive in my life. Walking toward the parking garage, I finally let go and my own tears flowed unabashedly.

A few years later, after a magnificent vacation in Bermuda, free of seizures and worry, I wrote this reminiscence in the form of a note to Graham. I would read it to him later, when the short days of winter seemed particularly bleak:

"Bermuda was the best, wasn't it, Bud? Lisa brought her husband,

Al, so we had all the muscle power and support we needed. Your mom prepared and froze your favorite meals. We had the big room at the Southampton Princess with its spectacular view of Riddle's Bay at sunset. Our greatest discovery was the little crescent beach next to Horseshoe Bay, which sparkled with pink grains of sand. Partially hidden by Sago palms, wispy Australian pines and sea grape trees, that beautiful stretch of beach was our special playground for an entire week.

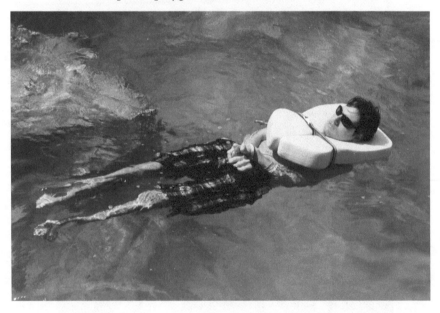

Bermuda was the best

"Every day, the air and the water reached the same perfect temperature: 83 degrees. Honeysuckle, morning glory and purple bougainvillea enveloped us in a canopy of tropical color and fragrance on our short trek from the hotel to the beach. There, on the south shore of the island, the ocean offered just enough of a rolling swell to make our swims interesting, without having to contend with big waves.

"We had our thatched hut to provide shade when we wanted

it, but you spent most of the day floating in that crystal clear, turquoise water, requiring almost no assistance from anyone. You bobbed alongside huge coral outcroppings forced up long ago by volcanic forces. At low tide, we saw thousands of tiny vertical marks on the coral left by the teeth of blue parrotfish feeding on algae.

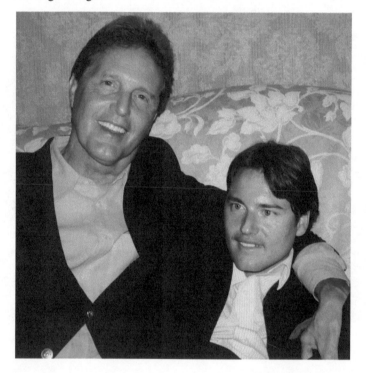

"You floated and relaxed. You were free. When you got a little chilled, we wrapped you like a cocoon in fluffy blue towels and let the sun warm you on your lounge chair. Lying next to you I experienced pure contentment, knowing that neither of us wanted to be anyplace else in the world in those moments. You smelled of salt and Coppertone. Your skin became beautifully tanned. You looked quite dashing in the green-and-blue plaid swimsuit your mom had packed for you.

"At the end of the day, after exchanging greetings with the hotel doormen in their pink shorts and black knee socks, we took luxurious hot showers and rested before dinner after rubbing our skin with lotion that made us smell like coconuts. After dinner, we had no responsibilities aside from watching the darkening silhouette of the Gibbs's Hill Lighthouse as the sun set over Riddle's Bay. We savored the gentle wind coming through the balcony doors and listened to the cheerful chatter of songbirds and the cricket-like singing of tree frogs. We talked, listened to music or read a book. And then we slept deeply, knowing we could do it all again the next day.

We were together in one of the most beautiful places in the world. Bermuda was the best, wasn't it, Bud?"

9

LIFE IS GOOD

When we were finally able to bring Graham home, to actually live in my house, *our* house, it was a euphoric time. Graham had been living, at least during the week, for a full decade at Crotched Mountain. He needed all the special help and services that were available to him there. But when a student turns twenty-two, "residential special education" ends. Families face a monumental transition as their children are required to move on. The resources that disabled kids receive are hard to find for young adults. Funding is limited and families often find themselves scrambling to find programs that assist with complicated needs.

After an aborted attempt to have Graham live in a group home two hours away from the area where we live, Cynthia and I sat down and figured out what it would take for Graham to come home and live with me on a permanent basis. It was intimidating, but possible. For starters, we would need great helpers and a qualified day program nearby. Destiny graced us when a one-of-a-kind individual materialized and agreed to assist us as Graham's primary aide. We found a day program called Bass River in the neighboring town of Beverly that was run by a compassionate and capable team. The building occupied by the agency was somewhat threadbare, but its staff were strong teachers and advocates.

And finally, Graham's special friend from Crotched, Lisa, agreed to come down and help us on weekends. In what seemed like a small miracle, all the pieces of our puzzle fell into place and, fittingly, at the start of the Christmas season, Graham moved home. He had a beautiful room on the ground floor of my house, with its own fireplace and filtered morning sunlight. He could see our big Christmas tree outside, adorned with colored lights from his bed. Cynthia helped organize and decorate the room to a perfection that Martha Stewart herself would have had to admire. Coming down the back stairs and finding Graham there on the first morning of our new life was an indescribable feeling. Graham was home. And so was I.

To transport Graham to Bass River for his day program, we discovered a service called the RIDE that allows disabled people to arrange transportation in accessible vans for a nominal fee. The drivers are good people who make sure that their clients travel safely from door to door. The very first morning that Graham traveled with the RIDE, I decided to follow it to Bass River, about a ten-mile trip. I wanted to see for myself how the van service worked and make sure that it was safe and comfortable for him. Graham was scheduled to be the only client in the vehicle that day. I pushed him down our driveway to the waiting van in his heavy wheelchair, bundled up in winter clothes. With a bit of trepidation, I watched the driver load him into the vehicle using a hydraulic lift. The man then carefully buckled Graham's chair down in the middle of the van, facing forward. I got in my Jeep and followed as they pulled away. I could easily see the wheelchair and the back of Graham's head through the van's rear window.

I experienced intense feelings on that frigid morning. There was a twinge of an old sadness that had to do with Graham requiring special services like the RIDE, with necessary, but somewhat dehumanizing, devices like hydraulic lifts. But, at the same time, I was grateful to live in a country where a service like the RIDE is even available and that it takes people with disabilities to programs where they are treated respectfully. Graham was an exceptionally handsome young man who was bright and good-natured. He would surely have been a shining star in our culture, if not for his disability. But his cerebral palsy forced him to rely on other people, sometimes complete strangers, for absolutely everything. And he accepted that assistance graciously and cheerfully.

Through my windshield, I watched Graham's head, covered by a black fleece winter hat, bobbing as the van hit potholes. At a traffic light, I wondered if pedestrians on the sidewalk simply saw a handicapped man in a van, glad it wasn't them or someone they loved. The person I saw was a human being of uncommon grace and dignity. Although I had always been hugely proud that Graham was my son, my heart was unusually full that day. Waiting for the light to change, I could make out a familiar circular decal stuck to the back of Graham's wheelchair. The sticker had been a gift to Graham from our friends Kathleen and Shawn, along with several T-shirts featuring an ever-smiling character named "Jake." Gazing through the rear window of the RIDE van on that frozen morning, joyful that I was Graham's father, the message of optimism on the shirts and decal rang true for me, more than it ever had before: "*Life Is Good.*"

When Graham was just a youngster, after California and before Crotched Mountain, I was introduced to a delightful personal care assistant from the Ivory Coast who had once taken care of Lorenzo Odone, the courageous boy who was the subject of the book and film *Lorenzo's Oil*. Fatou N'Diaye was a joyful woman with amazing strength packed into a svelte frame. She sometimes wore the colorful hand-painted traditional dresses and matching headscarves that were native to her West African heritage in the Ivory Coast and Senegal. She typically worked several jobs at a time to make sure that her son, Cyril, would have a higher education and opportunity as he came of age in America. As busy as she was, when Fatou met Graham for the first time, she felt "a quickening of the spirit," and she offered to help us. She and Graham had connected as soon as their eyes met. As much as her schedule allowed, Fatou joined us and challenged her new recruit, persistently urging him to work at his physical therapy and communication skills. Fatou assisted Graham over a period of about five years and shared many happy holidays with us during that time.

Although Fatou had become "family" to us, we gradually lost touch with her during the decade when Graham went to school in New Hampshire. As the years passed, we kept up sporadic contact, but, insidiously, our lives grew apart. One year, in the weeks before Christmas, I realized that I no longer even had a current address for the radiant person who had been there for us when we had sorely needed her help. As Graham neared age twenty-two, one concern dominated our conversations as Cynthia and I worked out the complex arrangements that would allow our son to move home. The key challenge was finding a qualified helper to take care of him in my house when I was at work. We needed someone absolutely reliable who also understood and believed in Graham.

Subliminally at first, I began to wonder what had happened to Fatou. I recalled vaguely that she had worked in a dialysis unit as a technician somewhere outside Boston. Combing through the internet, I made a list of all the facilities near Boston that performed dialysis and began to call them one by one, leaving cryptic messages for "Fatou to call Dr. Gardner." I was not even sure what last name she was using or, for that matter, if she was even in the United States. Two days later, the phone rang. It was Fatou, and she was working in a town near Salem!

After catching up with one another for a few minutes, I screwed up my courage and asked if she would consider quitting what she was doing to take care of Graham. It was a long shot, and I felt sheepish, embarrassed that we had lost track of her for so long. Fatou agreed to think it over. If nothing else, she would come over soon for a visit and a long-overdue reunion with us. On the appointed day, the doorbell rang, we shared a hug and Fatou came back into our lives. "Steven, I've thought about it, and I've decided I want to take care of Graham."

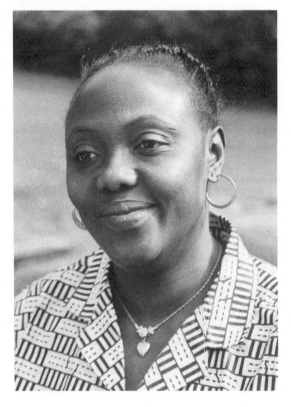

Fatou

It already felt like a miracle that Graham was coming home. We had found Bass River's excellent day program and reliable transportation to it. Cynthia had stocked our freezer with delicious frozen meals, spruced up Graham's room and updated his wardrobe. But we needed someone to get Graham going in the morning, get him settled at home after he returned from the day program, work with him on his physical therapy, feed him dinner, bathe him, get him ready for bed and be available to manage any unforeseen problems in my absence during the day. It was a big job.

Improbably, that unique person was someone we already knew. Someone who already cared for Graham. Someone with a knack for appearing at the exact moments in time when we needed her the most. Fatou! On the very first day of our new life, I returned from work to find Fatou and Graham singing in the bath. A shiver passed through me. It was the joyous realization that we were finally *home*.

Now that we had the key elements of Graham's daytime schedule in place, thanks to Fatou and Bass River, we had one more need to fill—someone to monitor Graham at night and to make sure he was safe while I was asleep. Fatou came through again. She had friends from Africa who did just that sort of thing and she volunteered to make some calls. Before we knew it, Kadiatou Barry, a tiny, graceful mother of three who had been born in Guinea, West Africa, rang the doorbell, gave Graham a warm greeting and asked when she could start. Kadiatou knew from Fatou how proud I was of my son. So she addressed me as "Baba Graham," (father of Graham), not "Doctor Gardner," and I loved my new name.

The job consisted of coming to the house at around 11:00 p.m. and making sure that Graham was okay until I woke up around 6:00 a.m. Usually, Graham would be sleeping during those hours, but Kadiatou needed to be ready to help him if he was awake and needed a drink or, more importantly, to wake me, in the event that Graham had a seizure or some other medical emergency. Kadiatou proved to be reliable and kind.

She was perfect in her role, and I slept soundly, knowing that Graham was being monitored with care.

Kadiatou sometimes dropped by on her days off just to check on us. I thanked her for her attentiveness and explained that Graham and I had a relatively small biological family and that the kindness we were receiving from our friends from Africa meant a great deal to us. Kadiatou looked at me and said: "Steven—you *never* are alone now. Graham make you have big family."

Sharda Desai was a vibrant powerhouse of a woman who had been an early women's rights advocate in her native India. She came into our lives in a random way when I was arbitrarily assigned to be her primary care physician at Massachusetts General Hospital. She was a robust middle-aged woman in excellent health, and I saw her for only a few relatively trivial issues over several years. Sharda was proud of her four children, including a son, Sai, who had been born some thirty years earlier in Mumbai with a congenital heart condition. As a child, he had undergone several surgeries and had done well for more than twenty years. But as a young adult, he had become progressively short of breath. A faulty heart valve needed to be replaced. He came to Boston for the surgery.

Sharda brought Sai to my office one day out of sheer maternal pride, and he was, indeed, everything she had bragged about. I sensed that he was a young man destined to make a difference in the world. About a week later, Sai underwent the surgical procedure at another hospital. After just a few days, he was discharged and taken to his mother's apartment near Boston. Later that same day, Sai collapsed in his mother's arms and died. His new heart valve had failed—spectacularly. In the weeks that followed, I tried to do what little I could to help Sharda in her grief. In the aftermath of that incomprehensible tragedy, I let her know that she could walk into my office without an appointment from that time on, and I would be honored to see her if she needed me. She was understandably shocked and angry.

On one of those visits, during a pause in our discussion of grief, Sharda looked around at the photos in my office and asked me to tell her about my own son. I confided to her that Graham was severely handicapped by cerebral palsy. The news surprised her because the photos showed the beautiful face of a robust-appearing young man with no visible hint of a disability. Something shifted in Sharda. She became visibly moved and said nothing for a little while. She continued to study the framed images of Graham and me on my desk. The tidbits of news I had previously shared with her about my son had communicated pride and happiness. She expressed surprise that there had been no bitterness or sadness in my voice.

A few months later, Sharda went home to India to be with her family. We kept in touch sporadically via email. She seemed increasingly curious about Graham, and asked for more details about his life. I was happy to tell her all about him and how joyful it was, for Cynthia as well as me, to anticipate having him living at home before long. After a period of time, Sharda returned to Boston from Mumbai. She phoned to say that she had brought us something, and I invited her to visit us. Graham was home by then, and he and I picked her up at the train station in Salem on a bitterly cold winter day.

After exchanging greetings and drinking some herbal tea, Sharda opened a heavy, oversized handbag which she had carried with her on the long flight from India. She carefully removed a remarkable statuette about ten inches long. It was a hand-carved mahogany elephant. Holding the gift up to Graham, she said, "An elephant is never unable to bear the burden of his tusks."

Turning to me, she said:

"An elephant is a symbol of quiet strength."

As I struggled to find the right words to thank her, she looked from Graham to me and said, "Even the poorest person has something to give, and the richest person has something to receive."

We placed the singular gift on our coffee table facing our front door, a talisman. In that moment, she became "Auntie Sharda" to Graham. A few days later, I received an email from her: "It is another beautiful day, Dr. Gardner. I pray that you may be sustained from above so that the life which depends entirely on your devoted care may never suffer want as long as life endures."

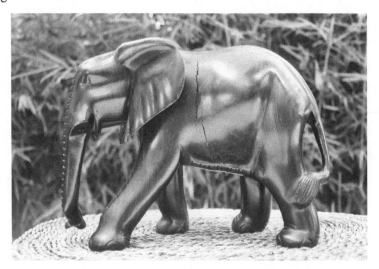

Talisman

It didn't take us long that December to begin thinking about the possibility of a very different lifestyle—somewhere warmer. Even as Graham was moving home during the Christmas season, we began to seriously consider moving much further south in the not-too-distant future. Our home was cozy, but outside it was dark, dreary and cold. We had always immensely enjoyed our spring breaks in the tropics, but that was one week out of fifty-two. Winter in New England is stunningly beautiful during a snowstorm. But maneuvering Graham's wheelchair on narrow sidewalks glazed in ice the next day was getting old for all of us, particularly when biting winds added to the struggle.

So we began to dream about a location that would be friendlier for us year-round, a place where Graham could be outside every day in shorts and a T-shirt. My mom had lived in South Florida for years, and I felt a connection with that tropical way of life. I loved the majestic banyan trees and the coconut palms that rustled in the wind along the beach. In contrast to the lifelessness of the New England landscape in winter, the luminous magenta of bougainvillea bushes and the vibrant pinks and yellows of hibiscus plants always seemed to lift the spirits. The massive afternoon formations of cottony cumulus clouds backlit by the setting sun were a stunning contrast to the never-ending gray of the opaque sky above Boston.

I met with a realtor in Delray Beach, and she showed me the ideal home for us. It was a Bermuda-style house on a breezy street lined with royal palms, halfway between the ocean and the Intracoastal Waterway. It had fragrant gardenia bushes, a pool and a little guest house I thought might be perfect for Fatou. The main house was small, but would suit us nicely.

Right across the street from the property was the waterway, where it widened out dramatically near a drawbridge—perfect for kayaking. At sunset, we could bike along Ocean Boulevard and watch pelicans glide and dive above the turquoise water of the Atlantic.

I didn't think it would be hard to find a job in Delray Beach, maybe even in a place where Graham could come with me—a day care center or a rehab facility. With Graham's magnetic personality, we would make new friends quickly. It would be a healthy life, lived outdoors to a great extent, free from the chilly confinement of winter in New England. Importantly, Cynthia loved the whole idea.

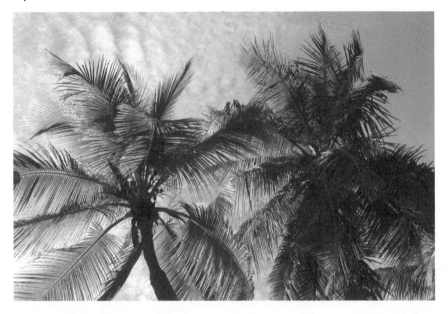

And, thanks to Google Earth, we could actually see the home we hoped to buy, and we began dreaming of that new chapter in our lives. In those dim days in the dead of winter in New England, it was delightful to picture ourselves in that sunny place, floating on the waterway, cycling next to the beach and watching the pelicans soar. And simply being together—somewhere warmer.

10

CHRISTMAS TREES

When I was an infant in Forest Hills, New York, in the borough of Queens, my mother supported us by modeling for the Ford Agency in Manhattan. Televisions were just beginning to appear in homes, and the visual media that people relied on were newspapers and magazines. Mom's innate elegance shone radiantly in ads for Saks Fifth Avenue and Tiffany & Co. in the *New York Times*, *Glamour* and *Vogue*. She was a fresh, natural beauty from a Quaker family in Bucks County, Pennsylvania, when she was "discovered" at age seventeen by a Manhattan model agency executive with a weekend home nearby. The lovely face that the agency director spotted was warm and unpretentious. Soon, Kathryn ("Kappy") Hobensack found herself on the covers of magazines for young women like *Mademoiselle*, to the delight and amazement of her family in the sleepy village of Doylestown. She shared some assignments in New York with an even younger beauty from the Philadelphia area named Grace Kelly, who was destined to become Princess of Monaco.

Over the years, Kappy's modeling assignments brought her into contact with other iconic personages of the day. She received a wink at the Stork Club from a distinguished gentleman at the next table who turned out to be Winston Churchill. And she was courted, albeit briefly, by the eccentric billionaire, Howard Hughes, who offered to take her to Hollywood, a notion that was summarily squashed by Hobie and Lavinia, Mom's unassuming parents.

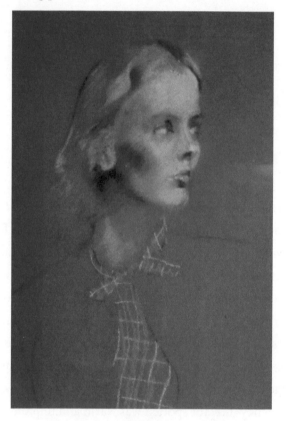

Mom during her modeling career

At the end of World War II, my father returned from Japan with what today would be termed PTSD. When I arrived on the scene, it was Kappy's modeling career that sustained our small family. While Mom worked in Manhattan, I spent my days with Anna Kohler, a rugged and kindhearted woman who lived with her husband, Al, in a tiny row house on Nansen Street in Forest Hills. Anna had desperately wanted a child, but was unable to conceive and there were no fertility clinics then. On some level, I became the answer to her prayers. Al looked something like Norton, the Art Carney character in The Honeymooners, and, like him, worked long hours as a plumber. He wore sleeveless T-shirts that were pungent, even to the inexperienced nose of a toddler. He and Anna bought me a surfeit of toys, including a miniature drum set, and stocked black cherry soda in an icebox in their little basement.

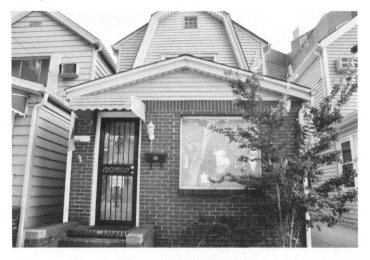

Anna's stoop

Anna happily doted on me. When Mom attended evening events in the city, Anna was overjoyed to have me spend the night on Nansen Street. She referred to me as her son when we passed people on our walks, a reference that led to some confusion and raised eyebrows among her neighbors. In the summer we sat contentedly, side by side, on her narrow brick stoop with Chickie, her curly-haired little dog, waiting for the joyful jingle of the Good Humor truck that brought us Creamsicles. I loved to ride the Nansen Street sidewalk, bumpy with tree roots, pumping the pedals of my shiny red fire truck under Anna's watchful eye. I enjoyed her "peasant" foods, like mashed carrots and potatoes, served on a classic 1950s chrome and formica dinette table. On chilly days, she gave me warm milk with sugar and a tiny splash of coffee. They were happy times for us both.

Anna was my nanny until I turned four, when Mom and I left for New England without my father. I have a dreamlike impression of her standing on the sidewalk of Nansen Street in a faded apron, stockings rolled into loops above her sturdy ankles, giving me a tearful smile as we waved goodbye for the final time. But it was not to be the final time. After more than two decades, Anna and I would be together again.

While working in Manhattan on a medical school elective in hematology, I picked up the ponderous New York City phone book on a whim and, with some amazement, found Anna's name. Implausibly, I recognized her four-digit Nansen Street address after all those years. Her warm voice was instantly familiar when she answered the phone. A few hours later, I boarded the subway at Lexington Avenue for the short ride to Forest Hills. On my short walk to Nansen Street from the station, the sights and sounds of the modest neighborhood were instantly familiar. I found Anna standing in her doorway in a state of quiet excitement. A widow now, she told me that, for more than twenty years, she had been praying that we would be reunited. On the spot, we decided that I would stay with her—in my old room—for the duration of my four-week rotation at Roosevelt Hospital.

For Anna and me, that unexpected time together mirrored the happy days we had shared so long ago, except that, instead of riding down the sidewalk in my firetruck, I took the subway into the city. In the evening, sitting together on her stoop, we were as happy together as we had been two decades earlier. A few months later, Anna attended my medical school graduation and said it was the proudest moment of her life.

My old friend and I talked on the phone from time to time, but I was soon swallowed by the all-consuming grind of my medical residency in Boston, and communication between us insidiously dwindled. As the years passed, preoccupied with getting married and starting an internal medicine practice outside Boston, I lost touch with Anna for the second time. However, out of the blue, perhaps three years after our last contact, I received a phone call from one of Anna's neighbors. She told me that Anna had developed Alzheimer's disease and was in a long-term care facility. Anna must have given the neighbor my contact information, but for some reason, she hadn't thought to call me sooner. That weekend I drove to a bleak, state-run nursing home on Long Island and learned from a kind Haitian nurse that I had been Anna's only visitor in nearly a year.

A few months later, the same nurse called to tell me that Anna had died. On an anemic winter day, I drove back to Long Island and was heartbroken at the sight of her burial plot—a haunting rectangle of dirt bordered by grimy snow under a clamorous, rusting expressway. The vast cemetery covered the landscape like a dingy gray blanket that seemed to stretch all the way from Queens to the East River. There had been no actual funeral, no memorial service, no celebration of her life. Anna had left no living family. In that desolate place, braced against a biting wind, I was stunned that such a lovely human being had left behind a mark so small that—beyond that rectangle of dirt and a tiny marker—it appeared to be almost nothing.

In that moment, I realized that the legacy of Anna Kohler—perhaps the only evidence that she had even lived on the earth—now resided in a *single* place—the domain of my own heart. I turned away from the grave and, without looking back, started driving north. During the drive home,

I tried to focus on my joyful memories of Anna and Nansen Street. It was the Christmas season then, and two powerful visual memories awoke in my memory from those years as a toddler in Queens. Both related to Christmas trees.

Impressionistically, I remembered tall, brightly decorated evergreen trees on Queens Boulevard. The Christmas lights were multicolored and brilliantly mesmerizing to a toddler just learning about Santa Claus and the story of Christmas. But I recalled, even more vividly, the little Christmas tree that sat in Anna's tiny foyer. It was at most three feet tall. Anna had decorated it with strings of multicolored glass candles filled with oil that bubbled brilliantly. When I saw it as a toddler, Anna's Christmas tree was the most magical thing I had ever seen.

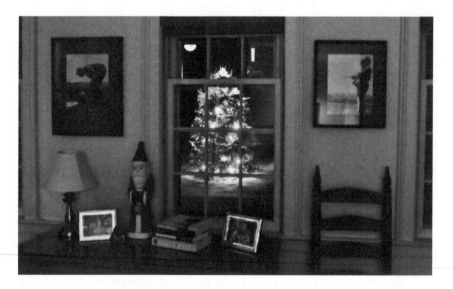

The Christmas tree from Graham's bedroom

Many years later, memories of Anna and those nostalgic childhood Christmas images awoke in me with surprising poignancy. Graham was home from Crotched Mountain, and we decided to begin a holiday tradition of putting up a big balsam fir Christmas tree in our backyard in Salem. It stood outside the rear windows of his room, where he could see it from his bed. We hung strings of big multicolored bulbs and waited for the first snowstorm, knowing that the snow would amplify the brilliance of the lights. Our backyard Christmas tree glowed in honor of Anna, and I wished that she had lived to meet Graham.

As Christmas approached, I decided to add a final touch of nostalgia to the holiday by finding a set of those glass bubble candle lights that I remembered so vividly from Anna's tree. We wound them around a small, freshly cut scotch pine tree in our living room and waited for the contents of the candles to warm. When the bubbles rose in the brilliantly colored candle-shaped tubes, I became a toddler on Nansen Street again for a few precious moments.

When Graham came home, I felt a happiness that was different than anything I had experienced before. It was Christmas time, and a real Tiny Tim lived in our home. In that season of hope and joy, I often thought about *A Christmas Carol*. Bob Cratchit said his fragile boy was "as good as gold. And better." And so was mine.

It had been a traumatic process figuring out Graham's transition, but we had. Cynthia was doing everything in her power to make it work. Our wonderful helpers brought a touch of the exotic to our house with melodic snippets of French, Spanish and even Swahili wafting from the kitchen. After a grueling stretch trying to sort out where Graham belonged, the perfect solution had emerged.

He was home.

Our eclectic support system was anchored during the week by Fatou and Kadiatou, with Lisa helping Cynthia and me on weekends, and

Auntie Sharda frequently checking on us by phone. At the end of the day, after Fatou left and before Kadiatou arrived, Graham and I were alone, father and son. But also kindred spirits who now shared a mysterious blessing—we had found a way to come home again. In his comfy bed, I would massage Graham's leg muscles before reading a story. I would kiss him one last time before turning out the light, putting up the side rails on his bed and turning on the audio monitor so that I could hear him from my room upstairs if he needed assistance. The future loomed happily ahead of us, full of possibilities not yet even imagined.

On Saturday morning, February 6, I heard him stirring at about eight o'clock. I went down and climbed into bed with him. It was about six weeks since he moved home. We dozed off together, with his left cheek resting on my chest and my right arm under his strong shoulders. When we roused for the second time, we made a decision to be lazy a while longer. We stayed in bed, and I read aloud from *Tom Sawyer*. The night before we had stopped at the place in the story where Tom and Huck witness the murder in the cemetery.

As I read, a gentle snowfall began, plump wet flakes drifting down languidly outside Graham's three rear windows. Periodically, buffeted by invisible puffs of wind, they would flutter and dance for a moment. Our Christmas tree, positioned straight ahead in the backyard, developed an icy frosting which made the lights glow with luminous halos. I had the sublime feeling that I was catching a glimpse of heaven. Graham was home and happy. I was happy. Cynthia was happy. At that moment, there was no place else on earth I wanted to be and nothing else I wanted to be doing. Lying there, reading and watching a gentle snowstorm next to my beautiful son was the perfect way to spend a winter morning in New England.

After a while, we got up reluctantly and I settled Graham in his wheelchair. I lit some candles and put on Christmas music, aware that we were substantially overextending the holiday season. But we were not yet ready to let it go. Still in our pajamas, we made banana pancakes and waited for Lisa to appear with her coffee and hashbrowns from Dunkin' Donuts. As always, she hugged Graham heartily and joked with him for a while as we prepared to leave for the pool at the YMCA. We all looked forward to the outing. Swimming combined therapy and fun for Graham and had been one of our favorite activities over the years.

Lisa and I packed Graham's swimming gear and towels, and off we went, filled with anticipation and pleasure, just as we had done scores of times together over the past decade. Walking from the back door to the Jeep, we passed the Christmas tree in the back yard and admired the lights as they sparkled brightly through the fresh snow.

There was nothing ominous about the day.

11

ANGEL IN THE SERVICE OF GOD

"May I feel your arms around me
May I feel your blood mix with mine
A dream of life comes to me
Like a catfish dancin' on the end of the line."
—Bruce Springsteen, "The Rising"

I was unprepared for what happened that morning.

Graham had endured hundreds of grand mal seizures in his life and come out of them all. Afterward, he was groggy and upset for a while, but he always came out of them. The seizure he had that morning in the pool at the YMCA seemed different from the beginning. Lisa and I were holding him in the waist-high water, surrounded by small children and their parents, when Graham's 120-pound body seized violently, and he began to vomit. I could see that he was aspirating stomach contents into his lungs, but I couldn't get him completely on his side (a safer position for his airway) without dropping his head underwater.

As we raced Graham up a ramp for people with disabilities in the cumbersome pool wheelchair we had left in the shallow water, Lisa and I simultaneously experienced a shocking sense of panic and dread that this time might be different. Racing from the pool to the nearby changing room where we could assist Graham, we watched in horror as his body became limp. He was turning blue and not breathing. We were in a narrow corridor next to the pool and had no choice except to press ahead to the little changing room. In that windowless room, my consciousness moved out of my physical body. I felt myself rise to a place in the ceiling or above it. In a dream state, I watched myself, fifteen feet below, lifting Graham onto the cold floor and checking for breathing and circulation.

Nothing.

I saw the tensed back of Graham's father in his wet bathing suit as he started CPR, while Lisa ran out for help. I saw that man push his breath into his boy's mouth and press frantically on his sternum. I saw that there was no response from the young man who was now lying there looking—although it was quite impossible—like someone who was dying. The man below me blew his breath more aggressively into the boy and pushed more violently on his chest. Graham had bit his tongue during the seizure and was bleeding. During mouth to mouth, his father had cut his lip on one of Graham's teeth. There was a moment in which the blood, the very DNA of a father and a son, merged in both mouths.

From the ceiling, I saw Lisa's growing horror as a lifeguard entered the room to assist with CPR. Someone appeared with a portable defibrillator, but there was no electrical activity taking place in Graham's heart, so the device was worthless. A group of burly EMTs arrived, looking out of place in their heavy boots and orange safety vests, and I saw Graham's exhausted father allow them to take over the resuscitation effort.

Suddenly, I was back on the floor of the changing room. The EMTs were taking Graham out to an ambulance. It was then that I realized how cold I was. It was a kind of cold that I had never felt before and have no words to describe.

Looking at the flashing lights of the ambulance in the driveway of the YMCA, I had no doubt that the EMTs would continue their ongoing exercise of advanced life support en route to the hospital. I had participated in scores of those desperate "code blue" situations myself.

But I already knew.

I had seen the lifelessness of the beautiful body and recognized it.

I had felt it.

The EMT's efforts would be in vain. The outcome was already determined.

Graham was gone.

Asystole (A-sis-toe-lee) or "flatline" is the complete absence of electrical activity in a failing heart.

I watched in horror as Graham was hooked up to the monitor in the emergency room at Salem Hospital and there was no electrical heart activity at all. He was not breathing on his own, either. In fact, he appeared to have died. A machine was breathing for him and a young man in green scrubs was performing compressions on his chest.

After about ten minutes, having received Lisa's emergency call, Cynthia arrived at the hospital. I led her into the terrifying, windowless room where our son lay, surrounded by a tangle of IV tubing, beeping monitors and total strangers. I watched her stand to Graham's left and cradle his head, speaking in a firm, clear voice directly into his left ear.

"Not this way, Bud. Don't leave us this way. It's not dignified for someone like you. Try to come back to us. We love you. Please try."

As she repeated those words with the stunning love and strength of a mother, the frenzied commotion of the code blue continued all around the table where Graham lay. His bathing suit had been cut off, blood was oozing from needle puncture sites and the ventilator was hissing into an endotracheal tube in his throat. A cardiologist had ordered another round of IV injections, including epinephrine and bicarbonate, in a desperate effort to stimulate Graham's heart. I watched the monitor over the table and it was a haunting, perfectly flat line.

Cynthia persisted. Strong, clear, loving words. "Come back to us, Bud. Give us a little more time with you. This is not the right way for this to happen for someone so beautiful."

And then—electrical spikes appeared on the monitor. It was impossible, but the flat line I had watched for so many minutes had been replaced by what looked like "normal sinus rhythm," the heart's normal pattern.

Graham's heart had started to beat again, on its own.

Unfortunately, severe damage had been done. While the heart's rhythm was back to normal, its pumping action could not keep up a normal blood pressure without powerful drugs. But, with those drugs, he had blood pressure and we were able to take him to the ICU. During that night and in the early hours of the next morning, it became clear that Graham's organs, including his brain, had suffered irreparable harm. Cynthia and I made the agonizing decision to turn off the machines and stop the medicines. We both knew it was the right thing to do. Graham would not have wanted to stay on earth in a vegetative state.

But, during those exquisite hours, we were able to talk to our precious son, hold him, massage his feet, kiss him and impeccably groom him. We shampooed his silky hair, shaved his beard, brushed his teeth and cleansed and moisturized his skin. We held his hands and spoke into his ears. For the millionth time, we told him how much we loved him and how proud we were to be his parents. His Aunt Mary Robb arrived from Pittsburgh and was able to hold Graham and be with us. Our devoted friend, Barbara, was there. Graham's steadfast friends and caregivers,

Lisa and Fatou, were with him. He was warmed by a handcrafted blanket given to him by a kind chaplain, Jane Kortin.

As a physician, by definition, I am a scientist. But I believe that Graham heard Cynthia in the Salem Hospital emergency room and decided to come back into his body so that we could be with him for those precious hours. Cynthia borrowed a pair of scissors and carefully cut a lock of Graham's auburn hair. She wrapped it with exquisite reverence in a piece of paper from a copy machine.

We thanked the nurses and doctors and left the ICU.

"Death ends a life, not a relationship."
—Mitch Albom, *Tuesdays with Morrie*

For many years I have exercised twice a week with a retired firefighter and former semi-professional football player from the hardscrabble town of Lynn, Massachusetts. After a distinguished career as a firefighter, Jason Connor became a sought-after personal trainer. Known for impeccable integrity and a wry sense of humor, he has a devoted clientele on Boston's North Shore. By his own admission, Jason was never a great student, especially when the nuns in his Catholic middle school tried to teach him six tenses of Latin verbs—he much preferred running in the open air of the playground. Notwithstanding his trials in school, Jason acquired a practical wisdom over the years and his clients today look to him not just for fitness training, but for help in rebalancing their lives. The white-haired Irishman can be nurturing or tough, depending on what he senses his patrons need on a given day. When I pressed him about a scrap of paper protruding from his pocket one day, he confided that the note said, "I am a source of comfort for those in need."

While I enjoyed a privileged childhood in a leafy suburb, Jason grew up on the mean streets of a city. How mean? According to his brother, when Jason was about sixteen, he was shot, stabbed and hit by a car—all in the same day! The story sounds apocryphal, but I happened to overhear Jason and his brother marveling about it, not long ago, and realized that it actually happened. I wondered how he had avoided being bitten by a dog that day. Jason and I respected one another as soon as we met. Over time we became friends and we have fun teasing one another about our cultural differences.

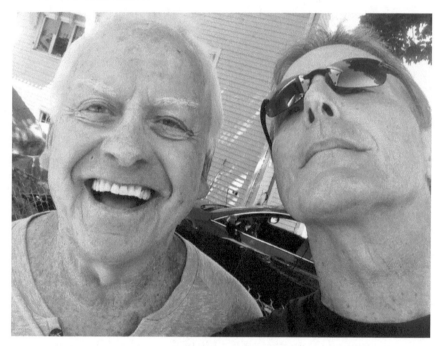

Jason and the author

During the training sessions, we lift weights, stretch, share corny jokes and talk about physical and spiritual goals. At the end of a workout, we meditate for a few minutes. During those periods of reflection, Jason has taught me to identify negative emotions and fears and to visualize myself dropping them into a wastebasket and pulverizing them, much the way you drag an item into the trash on a computer. Poof! He taught me to do just the opposite with the "good stuff." Drag my blessings to a place in the center of my consciousness where I can appreciate them more immediately and savor them. I leave Jason's feeling energized. As I take my leave, his final incantation is "Stay in the now!"

My friend had met Graham in our home and knew the details of his unique life and exactly what he meant to Cynthia and me. On the morning after Graham's death, the person I turned to was not one of my erudite comrades at the medical school, not one of my childhood chums and not one of the college schoolmates I love dearly. It was Jason. I drove to his house in a kind of trance. First, he cried with me. Then he suggested that we go through the motions of a workout before sitting down and facing one another to meditate.

I knew that I would never feel love so powerful again. I knew that the world would never be as wonderful as it was with Graham in it. I knew that I was in a state of shock and that my relationship with grief was only beginning. Unlike the relatively minor tribulations I had confronted while meditating with Jason in the past, I had no interest in putting this monumental tragedy in the trash and vaporizing it. I would never want to stop thinking about my son, marveling at the person he became and treasuring the life we shared.

Through tears, I looked at my friend and blurted out, "I'm not sure I know how to go on."

There was not a moment's hesitation from my friend who sat there placidly, an unlikely Irish version of Buddha.

"Take him with you," said Jason.

On one of our "spring break" trips to the Virgin Islands, a chambermaid at the Frenchman's Reef Hotel in Saint Thomas was smitten by Graham when she appeared to clean our room. Euthalie Daniels is a merry, freckled West Indian woman who has worked at the hotel for most of her adult life. When she saw Graham in his wheelchair, eating a meal with Lisa on our porch overlooking Charlotte Amalie Harbor, something stirred in her. For the next week, she couldn't do enough for Graham and the rest of us in his entourage. Euthalie impishly doted on Graham, teased him and made him laugh. We learned a little about her own life, teased her too, and got *her* to laugh.

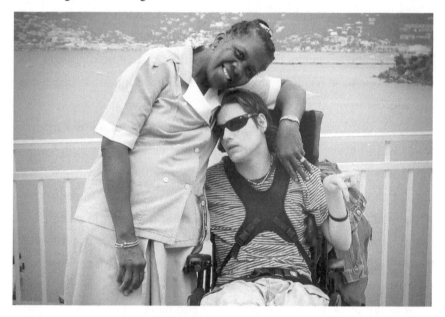

Euthalie and Graham

Watching Euthalie's big grin, I thought about how naturally Graham created bridges across cultural differences that frequently divide people. I had watched him do that for a long time. With Graham in our midst, those barriers simply didn't exist. We brought Euthalie a gift from New England when we returned to Saint Thomas the next spring. She presented Graham with a colorful polo shirt and some souvenirs. They both enjoyed the reunion. When we checked out to return home, Euthalie came to the hotel entrance to wish Graham well. There were hugs and promises to see one another again next year. But that was the last time we would see her. We decided to go to Bermuda the following year and never returned to Saint Thomas.

When Graham passed away, I sent Euthalie a note and thanked her for her kindness. She sent back her condolences and said she had worried when she didn't see us again. After reflecting on the instinct that drew her to Graham, Euthalie concluded by saying, "Try to be strong. Sometimes the best ones are taken away from us. Life is like that."

We were lucky to have a warmhearted young funeral director, Jason Fitzgibbons, to escort us through the unthinkable process of burying a child. Cynthia and I had already decided on cremation, and Jason handled those grim arrangements, along with the surreal, but obligatory, paperwork necessary to certify a death. The young man also assisted with the preparations for the celebration of Graham's life at Old North Church in Marblehead, the minimalist sanctuary where, twenty-two years earlier, Graham had been baptized.

Cynthia's sister, Mary Robb, helped us through each step of the numbing process at the funeral home. After the major decisions were worked out, Jason walked us through the chilling forms required by the Commonwealth of Massachusetts, impersonal pieces of paper that document the end of a life. Exact spelling of name, date of birth, date of death and—occupation? Mary Robb, Cynthia and I paused and looked at one another. Of course, Graham had never had a job in a conventional sense. (Although I had always thought that he would have been a perfect *model* for a clothing company interested in offering a different connotation— not just a beautiful *person,* but a beautiful *human being.*) Jason waited patiently, pen in hand, while the three of us considered the question.

"Well, he was an angel," said Cynthia.

Mary Robb and I enthusiastically agreed. If an angel was a benevolent celestial being who was a kind of intermediary between heaven and earth—that fit Graham nicely. If spreading love was an "occupation," he had been a highly successful entrepreneur in that line of work.

Jason was still waiting patiently.

"Absolutely—he was an angel," I said.

"An angel in the service of God," said his mother and aunt, in unison.

An uncertain look came over Jason's face, pen poised on the surface of the legal document.

"Do you really want me to write that down?"

"Yes."

And so Jason did. When the official death certificate from the Commonwealth of Massachusetts arrived in the mail a week later, the "deceased" was officially listed as "Graham Hale Gardner, Angel in the Service of God."

I decided to get back to work about three weeks after Graham died, hoping it would be a distraction to focus on other people.

At home, in the special haven we had created for Graham (and for me), I was haunted by the mementos of his remarkable life, especially the poignant souvenirs from our trips and adventures. It was painful to walk by ordinary objects, like the sneakers I set out for him to wear in the morning. Yet, it was too soon to put those things away. In my disbelief and grief, I knew I had begun to look for signs—anything to suggest that, in some form, our precious son was still here. Cynthia and I both, in fact, searched desperately for anything to fuel that hope. In those surreal days I began to notice RIDE vans driving next to me on the highway or crossing my street at intersections. Was Graham's path crossing mine? Was he sending a signal? My mind pictured the *Life is Good* logo on the back of his wheelchair that I had seen so clearly through the rear window of a RIDE van, just a few weeks previously.

Graham passed away on February 7. I had ordered a two-person tandem bicycle with a chair for him in the front that was to be delivered on March 4, his birthday. We had excitedly planned to begin training when the weather warmed up and ride again in the Pan Mass Challenge. In a kind of dissociated state, I listened to my own voice on the phone, numbly canceling the order for that special bike.

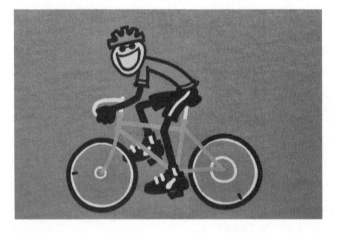

The thought of returning to work made me nervous. Surely, many caring friends and colleagues would be there for me. But I didn't want to be the object of anyone's pity. Over the years, my patients invariably asked me about Graham, having seen his photos all over the office. I would have to explain repeatedly what had happened and deal with the shock of those good people and accept their sympathy. But, after a while, I knew the time had come. With some trepidation, I walked into the clinic that first morning and accepted hugs from everyone. I slowly made my way back to my office and waited for the first patient of the day, a fifty-year-old man. He was seeing me immediately after a cardiac stress test, fifteen minutes of running on a treadmill while hooked up to an EKG machine.

He walked into my office, hand outstretched, still sweaty, wearing his clothes from the stress test—tattered gym shorts and a T-shirt. A blue *Life is Good* T-shirt featuring a boy on a bicycle with an ear-to-ear grin on his face.

"His soul had done what it came to do."
—Garth Stein, *The Art of Racing in the Rain*

Dr. Lewis Hays is a hospice physician who greets the world each day with an infectious grin above a salt-and-pepper beard, a loud bow tie and zany suspenders he refers to as his "braces." On a daily basis, he deals with the existential questions that arise at the end of human lives. From his life's work, this compassionate man has become convinced that human beings have much to say about how and when they pass out of this world. Over lunch, Lew shared this strong conviction about the end of Graham's life: "Graham needed to come home from Crotched Mountain, and then he needed to go."

I thought long and hard about that statement afterward. Lew knew that Graham's life had been an inspiration to many, and that he was cherished by an unusual number of people. But, no matter how much he was adored, Graham's life had also been a chronic struggle with muscle spasticity, seizures and physical discomfort. Lew believed that Graham had set a goal of making it home to live, and having accomplished that, he was ready to let go of the body that tormented him. He needed to free himself—and maybe his parents—from the confinement of his disability.

Barbara Pompea, a dear friend of Graham's and a constant source of support for us over many years, voiced a similar opinion. She felt that Graham did not want to get older in a body that betrayed him so often and did not want his parents to be restricted to caring for him for the rest of their lives. Wade Johnson, the Edgartown light keeper, believed that Graham "knew that his mission was complete" and that he was prepared to leave this world. I was grateful to those friends and respected their beliefs, but I wasn't fully convinced that Graham was "ready to go." Maybe what happened was simply an electrical accident that disrupted the wiring between his brain and his heart.

I was with Graham that morning, and I felt his contentment as we watched the gentle snowfall outside his bedroom windows from the warmth of a down quilt. I saw his smile when Lisa arrived to visit us. I felt his enthusiasm when we left to go swimming, as we had done so many times before. I *felt* that Graham was happy here, as much on that fateful day as any other. Graham knew how deeply he was loved. Cynthia and I had always hoped that all that love could make up for the indignities he had to bear because of his cerebral palsy—having to be fed, struggling with bowel and bladder function, having little control over his own muscles and being unable to clearly express what he wanted or did not want.

In medical parlance, Graham died of SUDEP ("Sudden Unexpected Death in Epilepsy"), which is poorly understood, even among seizure experts. Was what happened simply an electrical short circuit, or was there more to it? Was Dr. Lewis Hays right? I had to accept that I would never fully understand what happened that day. But one possibility was singularly hopeful.

What if—when Graham's cardiac arrest occurred—he saw something literally out of this world? What if he had a vision of a place free of disability and pain? What if he sensed irresistible serenity and peace in that place? And what if he sensed a love there even more profound than the abundant love that surrounded him in this world? Or—was it possible that Graham was already familiar with that place?

12

LESSONS OF LOVE

"I saw that you were perfect and I loved you. Then I saw that you were not perfect and I loved you even more."
—Angelita Lim

A long time ago, when Graham was just a little boy, I wrote a song called "Lessons of Love" for him on the piano, never imagining that I would one day recite it at the celebration of his life:

> *"I dream you're running*
> *I dream you're free*
> *But your time is coming*
> *And your gift will be*
> *Joy for this world*
> *Teaching us*
> *Hard lessons of love*
> *I heard you singing*
> *I saw you dance*
> *Bells will be ringing*
> *This is your chance*

Joy for this world
Teaching us
Hard lessons of love
So what do you say
Show what you can do
Do it your own way
No one will ever take this day away from you
When I hear you laughing
When I see you smile
I hope that God shares you
For a long while
Joy for this world
Teaching us
Hard lessons of love."

When I approached Old North Church on February 20, 2010, on a sun-splashed, exceptionally mild winter morning, there were people lined up on the sidewalk in both directions, patiently waiting to enter the sanctuary where Graham had been baptized. Inside, ushers were already moving the overflow of Graham's friends and neighbors, along with many people I did not even recognize, to the Sunday school room downstairs, where they would watch the service on a video feed. I wondered how a 22-year-old who had never spoken could pack a church with 750 souls, many of whom would later describe the service that day as a "life-changing experience."

Old North was filled with an aura of grace. The congregation seemed to share a sense that this young man—so delicate, yet so strong—had been almost too perfect for this world. The rays of light entering the nave through huge Palladian windows had a golden hue. On that midwinter morning, an ethereal warmth seemed to bathe the big chapel. The acoustic piano music and spare vocals of Neara Russell filled the majestic church with a quiet poignancy. Each remembrance by family and friends was singularly moving. A rendition of "The Weight" by a group of campers and counselors from Camp Jabberwocky, led by Graham's first counselor, Pete Halby, filled the sanctuary with the spirit of Jabberwocky.

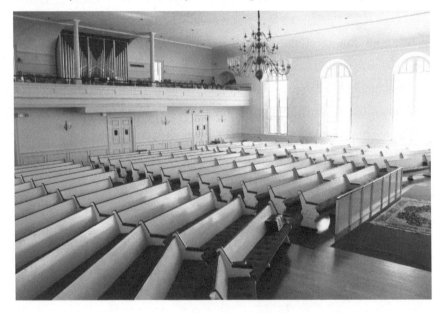

Old North Church

In those moments, Cynthia and I began to appreciate the magnitude of Graham's influence. It was not just a few dozen of our friends and family who had come out to support us. There were 750 people inside the church (and a handful still outside), and nearly every one of them seemed to have been affected by our son.

In the words of our friends, Sidney Morris and Margaret Knight: "There was a moment in the service after people began sharing memories, when we felt the room fill up with a presence that can only be described as love."

We carefully chose the songs that Neara Russell performed in Old North at Graham's service. Their melodies and lyrics spoke to our feelings for Graham and the man he had become. As a prelude, Neara played a simple instrumental piano piece I had composed myself called "New England Thanksgiving." Written in late November, I hoped that the song's spare quality and simple melody would convey a sense of gratitude for the blessings that we celebrate at that time of year, including the gift of having family to love. Hearing my own composition inspired by Graham's life, in the impossible setting of his death, was surreal but strangely fitting.

"Your Song," Elton John and Bernie Taupin's masterpiece, contained phrases and images that resonated powerfully for me at the triumphant time of Graham's passage home, including:

> *"Yours are the sweetest eyes I've ever seen."*
> and:
> *"I hope you don't mind*
> *I hope you don't mind*
> *that I put into words*
> *How wonderful life is*
> *While you're in the world."*

The haunting mood of Sting's "Fields of Gold" perfectly conveyed the staggering mixture of loss and gratitude we were feeling. In the precious weeks after Graham moved home, I might have told him:

> *"I swear in the days still left*
> *We will walk in fields of gold*
> *We will walk in fields of gold."*

Shawn Colvin's sentimental "I Don't Know Why" contained lyrics that seemed to allude to Graham and the other beautifully imperfect people with disabilities we had come to know and care about:

"I don't know why
But somewhere dreams come true
And I don't know where
But there will be a place for you."

It was Cynthia who suggested that we punctuate the service with a recessional hymn that would not leave people feeling melancholy, but would instead remind them that Graham had embraced life with an irrepressible sense of fun. The anthem Cynthia chose, "Take Me Out to the Ballgame," had always made Graham smile. While it might have been a surprising song to hear at the conclusion of a memorial service at Old North Church in Marblehead, it was a fitting finale for the celebration of an uplifting life.

Many friends of Graham and his family reacted emotionally to the memorial service. One friend, Katie Couric, then the anchor of the *CBS Evening News*, gave this beautiful remembrance in a broadcast two days later:

"I went to a memorial service on Saturday for someone who was twenty-two. Graham Gardner had cerebral palsy and died of a seizure and cardiac arrest on Super Bowl Sunday. He was swimming with his dad, one of his favorite things to do.

He couldn't speak and needed assistance doing just about everything. But he could swim and ski and windsurf, ride horses and kayak, often on equipment adapted for people who do things a little bit differently.

His mother and father, Cynthia and Steven, fiercely and passionately poured every ounce of their beings into giving their only child a life of joy and accomplishment. All who spoke, from his music therapist to his best friend, said he was a shining light who reflected all that love he absorbed. Graham showed us a life without limits, the strength of our differences, that kindness makes the heart fill up and flower. But it must be cultivated. And that's what the Gardners did, as a special and beautiful boy grew into an extraordinary man who embodied the power of love."

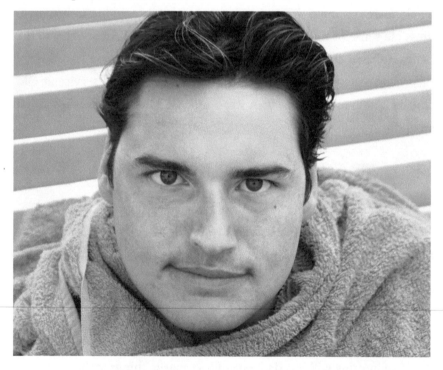

Graham's cousin, Mariel, was his soulmate, even though she lived in Pittsburgh and the two couldn't be together as often as they would have liked. The cousins were about the same age, and they formed a bond over the years that was based upon a communication all their own. They shared a mischievous sense of humor, too, that was unique to them. Mariel's mother and father describe her as an "old soul." At a young age, she had a spiritual nature and was more interested in existential questions than other kids her age. Very early in her life, she instinctively recognized Graham's inner light.

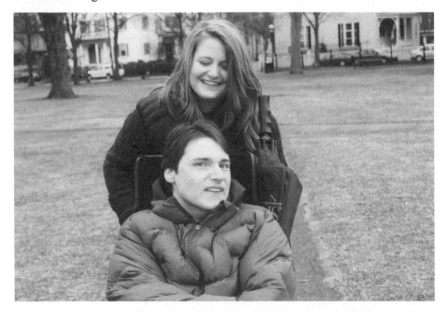

The cousins

When we were struggling to think of a catch phrase for the "memory card" that was to be given to the congregation at Graham's service, it was Mariel who immediately thought of the iconic phrase from the movie *Harold and Maude*: "Now go out and love some more."

Maude had uttered the remark when she was close to death and her young friend, Harold, was growing despondent. She told him that life was about renewal and hope. He must think in terms of new beginnings and, above all, he must never stop loving. Mariel had found the perfect message to honor Graham's legacy.

Earlier in that whimsical movie, when Harold told Maude that, of all the flowers in the world, he would want to be a daisy, she had asked him,

"Why do you say that?"

"Because they're all alike."

"Oooh, but, Harold, they're not. Look! Some are smaller, some are fatter, some grow to the left, some to the right, some have even lost petals.

You see, Harold, I feel that much of the world's sorrow comes from people who are *this*. (pointing to an individual daisy), yet allow themselves to be treated as *that* (gesturing to a field of daisies that all look the same)."

Maude's metaphor was not lost on Mariel and Graham. The cousins recognized and loved one another's uniqueness. At the service, Mariel, a strawberry blond beauty with knowing green eyes, said this about Graham:

> "From childhood, I have believed that Graham was born into his fragile body because his spirit was too strong and his soul was too good for this world. Although there will never be another angel quite like Graham, we must fill our hearts with the love he so selflessly gave us. By sharing that love, we don't have to imagine a life without Graham—he will always be with us."

Just four days before Graham, Lisa and I left for the YMCA, "Auntie Sharda" had written the words: "It is another beautiful day. We pray, Dr. Gardner, that you may be sustained from above so that the life which depends on your devoted care may never suffer want as long as life endures."

Neither of us could have known on that day that I would so soon experience the same unthinkable horror that had befallen Sharda. Now, in the raw early days of my own grief, it was my patient's turn to offer comfort. Her steady stream of emails contained words of sympathy, readings from scripture and, later, invitations to come and visit my "family" in India: "I cry with you as I continue to keep watch with you in the darkest hour. Dr. Gardner, your love for your son inspired me and helped start the healing process which helped me to once again embrace what remains of my life. You *will* find the strength to let Graham's spirit return to God, where it belongs. You *will* find in yourself the will to embrace your own life as it continues to unfold before you. Find solace in the knowledge that your son is at peace with the Lord as you read this and that someday you will be reunited with him in eternity with God."

13

THE BIG BUS

"There is a land of the living and a land of the dead and the bridge is love, the only meaning."

—Thornton Wilder

A short time after Graham passed away, an African woman whom I had never met phoned me. She introduced herself as "Your sister, Elizabeth." "Liz" had heard all about us through mutual friends in Kenya. Though a stranger, she had been sending me nurturing emails nearly daily in an effort to provide comfort in the days after Graham died. She knew how horribly I was grieving, and she patiently called back many times when I didn't answer her at first. When we finally connected, her voice was strong and infused with pure kindness. I listened for a long time. She spoke from a background of personal tragedy and emphasized the healing power of extended family—she actually considered me now to be her brother. She stressed the necessity of carrying on, as difficult as it seemed. She gently asked me to accept that I would never understand why Graham had been taken from us.

Elizabeth then gave me an intriguing metaphor:

"The One who created Graham thought it wise to take him back where he came from. In this world we are on a journey on a big bus, and when the bus reaches our home we must alight. Graham came to his stop. Baba Graham, you have been a bridge to bring Graham into this world. The bridge is there but the person who walked on it is gone. My prayer is that you will one day join Graham in the house of the Lord. You will both hold hands once more."

We spoke again a few days later. Consumed with despair at that moment, I asked, "Elizabeth, what if I want to get off this bus and look for Graham?"

"You can't do that."

"Why?"

"It is the bus driver who must stop the bus and let you off."

"Okay, Elizabeth, but who is this bus driver?"

"Your Maker."

In a letter that came a few days later, Elizabeth expanded her metaphor:

"The bus picks up and the bus drops off. It is not yet our time to be dropped off, but we must always be prepared, Baba Graham. Sometimes being on earth is like walking uphill on a very rough, rocky path full of thorns. Unless we look up to our Maker, we will not have peace on this journey. May He who makes the sun shine and rain rain give you everlasting peace, wipe your eyes and give you back your sweet smile."

Your Loving Sister, Elizabeth

When I returned to work, one patient after another comforted me in a poignant reversal of roles. I had decided long before not to be a doctor who keeps his personal experience completely off-limits to his patients. The majority of the people under my care knew exactly what Graham meant to his mother and me. I felt that the people I cared for could benefit more from our relationship if they knew something about my own life and my son's. That was especially true for patients who were struggling with adversity of all kinds, including grief and depression. I knew that I was a more *humane* doctor because of my experiences with Graham and other people with disabilities. Perhaps the knowledge that I had a disabled son made me more *human* in the eyes of my patients.

Some patients cried. Many offered hugs. Paradoxically, in a few instances, I found myself comforting them. Without actually meeting him, people from a variety of backgrounds had seemingly been touched by Graham's life. Dozens sent cards and made donations to our designated charity, the Bass River Day Program. I noticed immediately that some of the most extravagant gifts and donations came from people with very limited means. In my hour of grief, my patients turned the tables on me and gave me strength. And they continue to do so, even now.

After Graham's passing, one of those patients offered his heartfelt condolences while we sat at my desk in the clinic at MGH. Gazing at the extravagant gallery of photos of Graham in the little office, he looked genuinely grief-stricken. During the years I had known him, even though he was there to address significant medical issues of his own, the young man had never failed to inquire about Graham's progress. On that cheerless late winter day, that gentleman, who had three small children of his own, wanted to talk about Graham's life. Looking through a photo album, he noted that, in many of the images, Graham and I were in the water. One snapshot showed us in the warm therapy pool at Crotched Mountain. Another showed us swimming in Sunset Lake, at the base of the mountain. Other images had been taken at white sand beaches on Martha's Vineyard and in the turquoise waters of the Caribbean. In every picture, Graham and I were smiling.

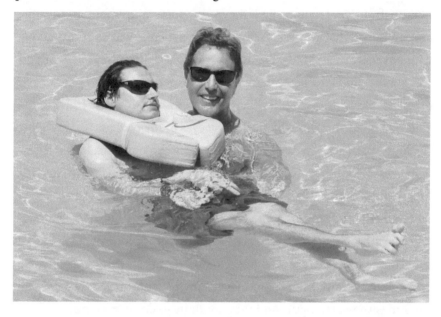

I told my patient that being in the water was soothing for Graham. The water's buoyancy allowed him to propel himself a little, without any assistance aside from the special life vest he used. It seemed to relax the spasticity in his limbs. In water, Graham was comfortable. In water, he had a measure of independence. My patient nodded. With emotion showing in his eyes, he looked across the desk at me with an expression of understanding. We moved on to other issues. A few days later, I received a hand-written note from him: "Doctor Gardner, I have been thinking a great deal about you since our conversation. I am so sorry for your loss. I want you to know that, in a very real sense, you were Graham's water. I hope *you* can find some comfort in that knowledge."

In the weeks after Graham's passing, my thoughts returned to Rabbi Kushner and the theological conundrum I had pondered a decade before. Horrific things happen to good people and, this time, the unthinkable had happened to us. But perhaps God's presence was evident in the extravagant response of our loving friends and family.

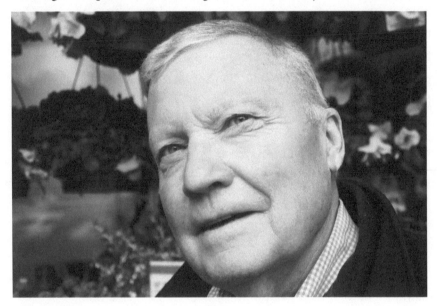

Frank

One of my supportive patients at MGH was Franklyn Shafer, a retired executive who surprised his family and friends by enrolling in a program in theological care at Boston University in his early sixties. The cheerful, rosy-cheeked gentleman became a hospital chaplain, a role that fit him perfectly. Spiritually curious and deeply kind, I always looked forward to seeing him on my appointment schedule, knowing that we would find time to squeeze in a provocative philosophical discussion about something going on in the world. During his first office visit after Graham passed away, Frank gently offered me his condolences. He had read Graham's obituary. We were pressed for time that day, but, as I was leaving for home, I found a note he had left for me at the front desk: "Graham was able to take in every bit of love from family and friends and magnify that love many times over and give it back in such a way that it could be recalled and passed on to others again and again."

Since he was in the midst of his theological studies at that time, I hit Frank with the Rabbi Kushner conundrum during his next visit. Can God be both good and omnipotent? We had a lengthy discussion about it in the office. A few days later, I received a letter from him containing this thought about Graham's passing: "Doctor Gardner, when that happened, I believe God was the first one to cry."

Several months after Graham's death, I was still struggling at work, hiding tears from staff and patients and trying hard to focus on the job at hand. Taking care of other people had sometimes been paradoxically therapeutic for me during times of distress in my own life. But this was more than distress. This was grief of the highest magnitude. I was startled by the haunted look of sorrow I saw in the mirror in the men's room.

On a particularly gloomy afternoon, I was listening to a hypochondriacal patient carry on in excruciating detail about some very trivial symptoms—he was sure that he was about to get a canker sore. My mind wandered to Graham as I glanced at a photo of him over the patient's shoulder. From my fifth-floor office, I allowed my gaze to drift down to Cambridge Street as the pallid light of another winter day faded. Young mothers hustled up and down the sidewalk pushing strollers. Cabs jockeyed for position in the chaotic Boston traffic. A firefighter polished a hook and ladder truck in the driveway of the station across the street. The routine elements of city life were carrying on normally, oblivious to the anguish I was feeling.

I closed my eyes for a moment, hoping the patient might think that I was pondering his troubling symptoms. In that moment, I subconsciously asked for help from Graham: *Bud, I am really struggling here. If you can feel me somehow, give me a sign and I will try to carry on. I could really use your help—right now.*

As I stared down onto Cambridge Street with that silent prayer in my soul, a vehicle stopped directly in my view. It sat there for ten seconds and then pulled away. It was a RIDE van.

My patient, "Helen O," was diagnosed with lung cancer ten years before Graham passed away. She courageously endured chest surgeries and debilitating chemotherapy and radiation treatments. Today, quite remarkably, she is considered "disease free." From my perspective as her primary doctor, Helen's resilience was amazing. She faced a terrifying illness bravely and never lost the faith that she could survive.

The first time I saw her after Graham's death, she offered me her condolences and told me a story that illustrated the ripple effect of Graham's life. Helen had been so moved by Graham's obituary in the *Boston Globe* that she gave photocopies of it to her friends. She had recently run into one of those friends who had, in turn, shared the obituary with his priest at a Catholic parish outside Boston. That priest, Father Joseph D'Onofrio, had then delivered a homily about Graham during a Sunday mass, despite never having met him. I decided to phone Father Joe to ask him what it was about Graham's story that inspired a sermon. He said that the obituary had brought him to tears and that he was moved by "Graham's ability to inspire people without saying anything in words." In his homily, Father Joe had described this as Graham's "paradoxical gift."

The young priest kindly met me at Saint Patrick's Church in Watertown, on the outskirts of Boston, on a splendid late summer day. He looked nothing like my stereotype of a priest, dressed comfortably in sandals, shorts and a T-shirt. It was his day off, and yet he sat with me in a sunny room in the rectory with a warm breeze blowing in through open windows and talked about Graham's "message." Father Joe explained that Graham's story confirmed for him that our spirits have essentially nothing to do with our bodies. He referred to the passage in Corinthians about faith, hope and love. I told Father Joe that I had 100 percent hope that I would see Graham again, but less than 100 percent faith, although I wished I did. He gave me a kind look and said that he understood. Although we had just met, we sat quietly for a couple of minutes in the sun-splashed room with tears in our eyes.

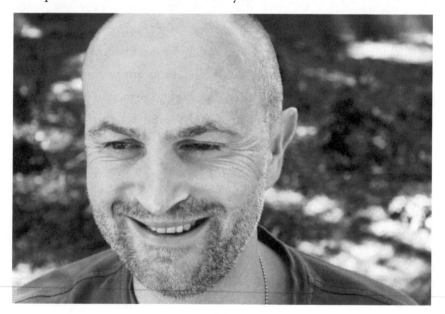

Father Joe

The idea that Graham was "an angel in the service of God" had resonated powerfully with the young priest. I mentioned that we had been amazed to receive about 1,500 condolence cards and notes after Graham's passing, obviously many from complete strangers. I showed him a note from "Jennifer," who had written to us after seeing the obituary, describing Graham as a "vessel full of divine life." Father Joe told me that his homily had explored that exact idea. Something inside Graham had radiated love—in a way that words often cannot.

A short time after Graham passed away, Cynthia and I attended a movie premiere and fundraising party for Zeno Mountain Farm, then a fledgling camp near Sugarbush, Vermont, for people with and without disabilities. Zeno now runs camps in summer and winter and creates films that feature all kinds of people. Their filmography includes a musical, a pirate adventure, a time-travel saga and several westerns that have received rave reviews at movie festivals. Zeno's ethos is "to be a catalyst for lifelong friendships—while being creative, thoughtful and present." The beautiful campus in the Green Mountains, complete with accessible tree houses, was created by Pete and Will Halby and their wives Ila and Bridget.

Pete, Will and Ila are Jabberwocky alumni and were among Graham's first counselors there. They cared deeply for him and were instrumental in introducing him—and his parents—to the intense kinship and zany fun that abound in communities like Jabberwocky and Zeno. Zeno features an accessible "swimming pavilion" built in Graham's honor at a pond on the property. Cynthia was instrumental in shepherding the project from dream to reality. She also joyfully volunteers as a cook there, in all seasons.

On the night of the fundraiser at the West Newton Cinema, just outside Boston, we joined a large, clamorous gathering that included friends from both camps. In our time of acute grief, it was wonderful to be back among those joyful people. The lobby was packed with campers and counselors along with their loved ones, a group that now felt like a second family to us. While Cynthia and I were heartbroken that Graham was not right there with us, we shared a powerful gladness that we had been blessed to be his parents and, through him, to be exposed to passionate and resilient people like the ones in the theater that night. Many of them were seeing us for the first time after our son's death and reached out to us with kindness and love.

As the exuberant group milled about before the premiere, chatting and laughing, Cynthia and I spotted campers in wheelchairs we had grown fond of over the years. Visiting with them, we subconsciously grasped the handles of their chairs. As I caught a glimpse of Cynthia playfully tipping back a camper and laughing with him, I experienced a strange epiphany: Cynthia and I missed pushing a wheelchair.

That sometimes burdensome aspect of caring for a disabled loved one now felt like something we had lost. For over twenty-two years, we had lifted Graham's heavy chair in and out of cars, pushed it down jetways and fought to maneuver it along icy sidewalks. It had been cumbersome and strenuous at times, and more than a few curses had escaped our lips over the years after scraping our shins on the chair's protruding metal parts. But the fact that the wheelchair held our son had made the device something very nearly sacred to us. At times, pushing Graham had felt like chauffeuring a prince around an unforeseen kingdom that contained magical lands like Camp Jabberwocky and Zeno Mountain Farm.

So we asked a few surprised parents if we might push their sons and daughters around the foyer of the theater for a little while. The rubbery handlebars felt familiar and comfortable. The weight of the occupied chair was easy to manage with coordinated movements that had long ago become second nature to us. It felt good to lean in over the backrest and rub a head, moving once again in unison with a very special person.

On a dreary evening in March, Cynthia bundled up against the cold and went for a walk at dusk. In her grief, she was numb as she walked past the stately weathered homes overlooking Marblehead Harbor, thinking about Graham. In a park she often visited with her son, she looked down absently and saw an object on the ground. She picked it up and recognized that it was a plastic scapular about two inches long. On one side was an image of Jesus and on the other was a likeness of Him with Mary. A tiny attached card read: "Now and at the hour of our death, immaculate heart of Mary pray for us."

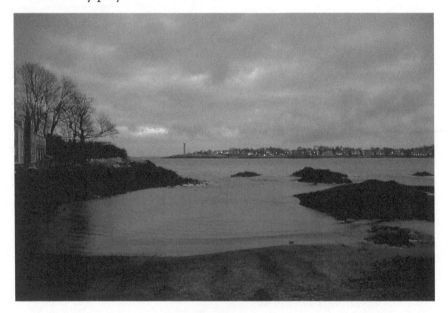

Marblehead at dusk

Devotional scapulars are carried as a pledge to follow a particular path, a reminder to the carrier to keep spiritual promises. Cynthia had no way of knowing what kind of pledge had been made by the owner of this particular scapular or whether his or her promises had been kept. But finding it in the aftermath of Graham's passing seemed serendipitous to her. After Cynthia showed me the scapular, I thought about the notion of immaculate hearts. Not many people have them, but Graham did. He was spiritually pure. As I thought about Cynthia's stumbling on the lost scapular, something began vaguely resonating in my mind—a passage from *The Prophet* by Kahlil Gibran that my mother had read to me as a child. The details eluded me at that moment and I went home to find the book.

I kept mom's copy of *The Prophet* in the drawer of Graham's night table, and I had read it to him not long before he died. I sat down with the book and found the essay I was looking for:

> *"Your children are not your children.*
> *They are sons and daughters of Life's longing for itself.*
> *They come through you, but not from you.*
> *Though they are with you, yet they belong not to you."*

Had Graham come through us into this world carrying a spiritual promise? I thought so. His promise, I believed, was to teach us about love. And, more specifically, to remind us of a conviction that he shared with Kahlil Gibran: "Beauty is not in the face—beauty is a light in the heart."

> *"The first premise of faith is to believe that there is*
> *no such thing as happenstance."*
> —Hasidic Aphorism

After the incident on Cambridge Street, when I asked Graham for help, I began to notice RIDE vans with an unlikely frequency. In my car, whenever my thoughts turned to Graham, it seemed that I would instantly spot one of those familiar, boxy vans with the blue and yellow stripes. Sometimes they would pass me, moving in the opposite direction. Sometimes they would cross my path at an intersection. Sometimes they would appear in front of me and parallel my way for a while before turning off. I wondered.

A patient gave me a thought-provoking book called *Invisible Lines of Connection*, in which Rabbi Lawrence Kushner asserts that there are no coincidences. I didn't remember seeing RIDE vans in the past. Maybe they were always there and I just didn't notice them. But now I was seeing them in a pattern that seemed to defy statistical probability. My drive to work required me to pass the YMCA where Graham's cardiac arrest occurred. Each day, I felt its looming presence on the top of a hill to my left and a sick feeling engulfed me until I was well past it.

One early spring morning, I shocked myself when I glanced up at the building and cursed it violently. I raised my left fist in a vulgar gesture at the same time. For that split second, I could make out the menacing structure on the hill and the blurred shape of my fist in the foreground. But something else was moving between the two images. A blue and yellow van had just passed me in the opposite direction and had literally come between my profane gesture and the building on the hill. The confluence of my angry outburst and my fleeting visual impressions—a building, a fist and a van—occurred in a fraction of a second.

I tried to calculate the probability of a RIDE van—, traveling forty miles an hour in one direction—and my vehicle—, traveling forty miles an hour in the opposite direction—passing one another in that uniquely intimidating location at the exact moment of my emotional eruption. The odds had to be vanishingly small. Pure happenstance? Or was Graham telling me not to despair?

My mother, "Kappy," weathered the unexpected storms of her lifetime with grace and equanimity. There were marital and medical crises that left her suddenly alone, and yet she did not complain. Under duress, she found joy in teaching music. She simply carried on and never lost her dignity or the ability to find comfort in friendships and the beauty of the physical world around her. Wherever Kappy lived, from New England to Florida, and places in between, she found it remarkable that a graceful, slender-tailed bird, the mourning dove, was always in a tree somewhere near, seeming to offer her a message of peace.

For Kappy, the mourning dove's cooing, like life itself, was simultaneously sad and hopeful. Its song had both a suggestion of regret and a promise of renewal. Before her death, she wrote this poem:

> "*Whenever I have wandered*
> *through places I've called home*
> *At break of dawn on quiet air*
> *The mourning dove was always there*
> *And when my life on earth is through*
> *My soul at rest in leafy glen*
> *The mourning dove will be there too*
> *With sweet, sad song*
> *and soft Amen.*"

Graham and I chose the Virgin Islands for one of our first "spring break" vacations by design. I had lived in Saint Thomas as an infant with Mom, when she was going through the painful process of divorcing my father. Throughout my life, I have cherished a Kodachrome snapshot she took of me at that time, swimming with another toddler at one of the world's most beautiful beaches, Megans Bay. Sentimentally, I wanted to go to that place with my own son, to experience the same tropical images and scents that Mom and I had shared a generation earlier. Going to Megans Bay became a kind of pilgrimage for us, a way of honoring the legacy of Graham's grandmother. Kappy was always happiest when walking a beach with sand between her toes. So we arranged to hire a wheelchair van to take us to the world-famous bay for an outing toward the end of our vacation week.

We were staying at Frenchman's Reef, the big resort perched on the cliff at the mouth of Charlotte Amalie's harbor where we had been befriended by Euthalie Daniels. Amy and Lisa, Graham's aides from Crotched Mountain, were helping us that year. We had breezy rooms overlooking that breathtaking inlet from the Caribbean. On the second or third day of our stay, I was feeding Graham his dinner on our balcony in the balmy twilight. There was a pleasant rustling of palms just below us as we watched a captivating parade of boats and seaplanes moving in and out of the harbor. Graham was having dessert when a mourning dove landed on the railing of the balcony no more than three feet from us. To our surprise, she perched there for no less than thirty seconds before flying away.

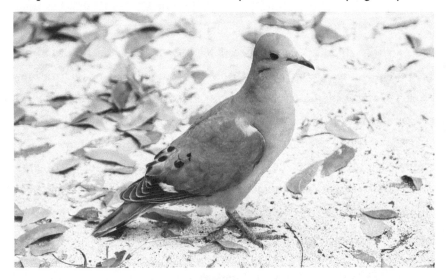

At Megan's Bay

The very next day, we made our excursion to Megans Bay. After swimming in the astonishingly clear, turquoise water with Amy and Lisa, we decided to rent deck chairs and relax next to a sea grape tree. It was the precise spot where I imagined Mom had snapped the old Kodachrome image. As the sun dried our skin, I sensed movement behind Graham's chair and looked around. A mourning dove with a patch of iridescent purple highlighting its beige plumage seemed to watch us for a moment before walking slowly away.

After Graham moved home, we occasionally heard the doves' song high in the trees on walks around Salem and Marblehead. But I noticed the birds with particular poignancy on an occasion about nine months after Graham passed away, during a humanitarian assignment I had accepted in Haiti following the devastating earthquake of 2010.

Years earlier, I had volunteered to be part of MGH's Global Disaster Response Team, but I had never actually been deployed overseas while Graham was alive. In his absence, I felt free to take the three-month assignment under the auspices of the international relief organization, Project Hope. When I arrived in Haiti, I found it hard to describe its heartbreaking squalor in words. Any understanding of the place was visceral—*smelling* the stench of festering garbage and latrines, *seeing* crumpled buildings that encased corpses and *hearing* the laughter of naked children innocently playing in the filthy water of sewage ditches. The atmosphere of hopelessness was hard to escape, even for the most hardened of the relief workers in our medical tent in the largest of the refugee camps.

About five weeks into my deployment, on a sultry night, a supervisor asked me to check on a French colleague who had become progressively ill at a darkened house in Port-au-Prince. As usual, the city's power was out, but my improvised evaluation—done by flashlight—suggested that Melanie, a veteran French humanitarian worker, though still in her early twenties, had cerebral malaria, a life-threatening form of the mosquito-borne disease. My instinct was that the petite powerhouse who had been a women's rights activist in some of the poorest places on earth would die if she stayed in Haiti. Her team leaders and I made the decision to transport her in a Learjet air ambulance from Port-au-Prince to Jackson Memorial Hospital at the University of Miami.

In the half-light of dawn, we flew over Guantanamo at the eastern tip of Cuba and crossed the Straits of Florida on the short flight to Miami International Airport. A waiting ambulance raced us to the hospital. After a flurry of tests and consultations with several renowned infectious disease specialists, we started Melanie on an aggressive combination of antimalarial drugs. She was awake and able to respond to questions, which was a good sign. That evening, I left her in the care of the hospital team and collapsed in a state of exhaustion at an upscale hotel on nearby Miami Beach. The elegance of the art deco tower was a startling departure from the wretchedness of Haiti.

I was worried about Melanie. But I was also worried about myself. The month in Port-au-Prince had been grueling and disheartening. Lying in the surreal luxury of a king-sized bed seemed like a moment that called for some soul searching. But I was sound asleep before my brain could think any more. In the morning, disoriented after a fitful sleep, I couldn't shake a gnawing feeling of loneliness and uncertainty. With Graham gone, I was adrift, anchored by neither parents nor children. I took a shower and dressed in the only clean clothes I had, a spare scrub suit I had brought in my backpack on the flight from Haiti.

Before the short ride to the hospital to check on Melanie, I sat in the hotel's opulent outdoor patio in a state of profound culture shock and ordered breakfast. It had been a long time since I had last eaten anything besides energy bars that tasted like flavored cardboard. I called the nursing station at Jackson Memorial, and a nurse told me that Melanie was better. While I waited for my breakfast, a family of three appeared on the terrace. The parents were speaking German and laughing as they pushed a boy in a wheelchair. He appeared to be about eighteen years old and seemed to have a permanent grin on his face. The physical features of his spastic cerebral palsy were very similar to Graham's. I was transfixed, watching the devotion of the parents and the boy's apparent happiness.

Watching bus boys discard untouched breakfast meats and croissants—just a day removed from treating people who were actually starving—was profoundly shocking. My brain couldn't quite fathom it and started to play tricks on me. For a few moments, the young man in the wheelchair actually seemed to have *become* Graham—except that he had a new set of parents who spoke German. Coaxing my thoughts back to reality, I watched the family closely. Their every movement and gesture were instantly familiar. I could easily sense the father's next move before he made it—positioning the boy in his chair, wiping his mouth, stroking his head. Every cell in my body could *feel* the aura of love that surrounded the boy and his parents.

Seeing that family should have made me extremely happy. But on that strangest of mornings, befuddled by exhaustion and grief, seeing them did *not* make me happy. If anything, it increased my sense of isolation and I had to look away. For the first time in my life, I wondered if I had lost my sense of hope.

As I turned away, feeling profoundly alone, I spotted the pair of mourning doves perched quietly on the terrace railing about ten feet away.

14

RETURN TO JABBERWOCKY

Returning to Camp Jabberwocky in 2010 loomed like an emotional impossibility, after so many years of magical experiences there with Graham. Yet, it seemed equally impossible *not* to return. The spirit of Camp had nurtured us over the years and the beauty of Martha's Vineyard had inspired us during some tough times. Camp Jabberwocky would surely be the one place on earth that would provide comfort in a time of unspeakable grief.

So, I decided to go.

Cynthia had been battling the same dilemma and arrived at the same conclusion. In fact, she had already made the decision to go and help with the cooking, a big job when there are as many as seventy hungry souls to satisfy three times a day.

The start of a new Camp session is cause for unbridled happiness and celebration. We didn't want to cast a shadow over that joyous kickoff, but everyone in the Camp family knew that we needed to mark the start of the summer of 2010 with a tribute of some kind to Graham. The first post in that summer's Jabberwocky blog had already featured a remembrance that was dedicated to "Graham, our friend and brother." As the campers and counselors began arriving in Vineyard Haven on a fine June day, Kaitlin Burkle, one of his most devoted counselors, had already conceived a plan for a celebration of Graham's life. After the campers had a chance to get settled, all of Jabberwocky gathered at State Beach, the special spot on the island's northeastern coastal barrier where the camp has congregated for more than half a century. In the clear twilight, we could make out Cape Cod across Nantucket Sound on the horizon. A few evening stars appeared. Graham's Camp family clustered close together at the water's edge, joined by some of our dear friends from the island. A few of us shared remembrances, including Kaitlin.

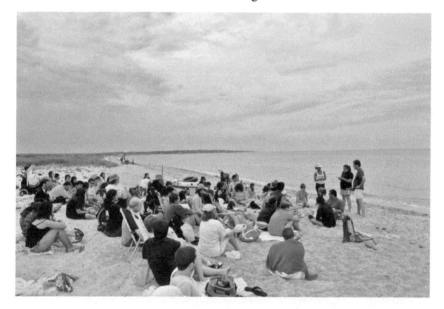

Kaitlin's remembrance

Campers who were able to do so waded into the gentle surf with Cynthia and me, leaning on one another for physical and emotional support. As the sun set, we scattered some of Graham's ashes in that sacred water. For a long time there was perfect silence, except for the gentle lapping of water caressing us with the incoming tide. Camp Jabberwocky, normally so wonderfully cacophonous, was stunningly still. During those solemn moments, Kaitlin and the rest of the counselors and campers released hand-painted paper boats into the water. They had stayed up half the previous night designing those singular works of art, each about five inches long. Although there appeared to be an onshore breeze that night, the fleet of paper boats sailed off gracefully to the northwest and disappeared into the darkness of Nantucket Sound.

Cynthia and I continued to look for signs from Graham. We yearned for a signal of any kind from our beloved boy. My brain had been trained to think in scientific terms. If Graham's spirit was around us in another form, part of the energy of the cosmos, would I have the capacity to recognize it? If his life force had merged with the inscrutable movements of the universe, would I be able to feel it? I wondered if I was too confined by "evidence-based thinking" to discover Graham in a new form.

I looked up at the scrub oak trees that form a canopy over Camp Jabberwocky. Was Graham up there in the wind rustling the treetops? Or in the subtle scent of the beach roses along the path to the Edgartown Lighthouse? Or in the powerful waves breaking on South Beach? For the first time in my life, I thought seriously about reincarnation. Could it be that Graham had entered the body of a newborn somewhere far away, starting life anew in a different vessel? If so, how would I ever meet him? And, if I did, would I know that it was Graham?

There was also another possibility—my ruminations about seeing Graham again were pure nonsense, time-worn fantasies intended to provide a bit of comfort for those who grieve and nothing more. Perhaps Graham was simply gone and never coming back. No longer here. End of story. As Cynthia and I struggled with that existential angst, we realized that the people of Camp Jabberwocky were becoming something more than summer acquaintances and friends. They were a much-needed extended family and source of comfort.

After experiencing the unforgettable service at State Beach and watching the paper fleet sail into the night, Cynthia and I ate supper at Camp. We visited until nearly midnight, as the counselors finished their preparations for the day ahead and the campers settled into their cabins. The unique rhythms of another year in that enchanted place were beginning once again—this time without Graham. Exhausted, Cynthia and I walked slowly down Greenwood Avenue toward Vineyard Haven. The familiar five-minute walk to Whiffling was cloaked in total darkness that June night. Our feet kept us connected to the stretch of sandy blacktop we knew by heart, but neither the moon nor a single star was visible. It seemed unusual that no light shone from any of the homes on that stretch of road. The sky was an impenetrable black dome above us.

After shuffling along for a minute or two, we began to discern tiny shapes moving in the darkness that cloaked us. A moment earlier, we had been immersed in inky blackness, but, suddenly, luminous flashes of light encircled us. Cynthia and I simultaneously realized that we were surrounded by literally hundreds of fireflies. This was a phenomenon that neither of us could recall during our many years on the island. In fact, we had never seen so many lightning bugs at one time—anywhere. Was Graham sending us energy and light, telling us that he would continue to show us the way if we could just be perceptive enough to recognize him in a new form?

At the memorial service for Dr. David Reid, Graham and I had been moved by the Hopi Prayer that his family had included in the celebration of his life. Among the fireflies on Greenwood Avenue that June night, as Camp Jabberwocky prepared for a summer without Graham, I thought about the prayer and found solace in its message:

"Do not stand on my grave and weep
I am not there. I do not sleep.
I am the diamond's glint on snow.
I am the sunlight on ripened grain.
I am the gentle autumnal rain.
When you awaken in morning hush,
I am the soft uplifting rush
Of quiet birds on circled flight.
I am the soft stars that shine at night.
Do not stand at my grave and cry
I am not there.
I did not die."

The day after we released the paper boats into Nantucket Sound, Camp Jabberwocky returned to State Beach on a glorious June day that was warm enough for sunning and relaxing in the sand. Everyone enjoyed the first cookout of the summer, featuring hot dogs, veggie burgers, potato chips and watermelon. The heartier campers and counselors braved the still-chilly water of the Sound and swam or floated on inner tubes out to a sandbar fifty yards offshore. The group out there was linked together like a ring of skydivers, holding onto one another protectively while splashing and teasing one another mercilessly at the same time. Meanwhile, at the water's edge, a more placid group sat in beach chairs, cooling feet that are often squeezed uncomfortably into orthotic devices. Some were catching up on one another's news of the last year and others were making new friends at the start of their very first camp session. Far back from the water, at the edge of the dunes, was a cluster of empty wheelchairs, happily vacated when their occupants were carried down to the water from the spot where the wooden ramp from the road ends.

Testing the water for the first time that year with my own astonishingly white toes, I noticed that a camper named Jamie was having a rough day. He had autism and looked anxious and a bit manic. His pacing back and forth in the wet sand at the water's edge seemed to mirror the motion of a few plovers who were pecking for food while darting in and out of the surf in their timeless dance with the waves. I watched Jamie bend down abruptly, pick up an object and inspect it for a moment. Something sparkled in the sun. His mood seemed to brighten as he handed the item to JoJo, our camp director. JoJo, whose exuberance cannot be quantified by any known scientific—or paranormal—algorithm, handed the object to me and, in a voice chronically hoarse from joyously yelling at everyone, said: "Look at this, Dr. Steve! It's a heart! Why don't you keep it as a memento of our love for Graham?"

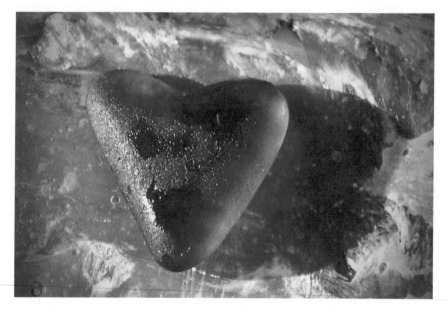

The heart

I took the tiny piece of glistening brown beach glass from her, held it up against the sun and marveled at its dark amber color and the smooth texture that had resulted from the relentless buffing of sea and sand. But the stunning thing about the object was its shape. It was, indeed, a perfectly shaped heart. It then dawned on me that Jamie had found the object in the exact spot where we had gathered for the celebration of Graham's life the night before. His finding it in that special place seemed serendipitous, even transcendent, and I wanted Cynthia to share in his discovery. On the way back to Camp, I stopped at a favorite shop in Vineyard Haven called Beadniks, bought a little red box and placed the heart in it.

Cynthia and I had a celebratory outing in Graham's kayak planned for the next day. I hid the box in my pocket with the intention of presenting the heart to her out in the Vineyard Haven harbor, the place where Graham had come and gone so many times with us on the big ferries with lyrical names like Sankaty, Katama and Island Home.

I had no particular plan as we paddled among the scores of graceful, moored boats on a calm, sparkling morning. It was wonderfully quiet in the middle of the harbor, our tranquility disturbed only by the cries of a few seagulls and the pleasant pinging of the rigging of sailboats. The gentle dripping of water off our paddles was interrupted once or twice by the startling but familiar blast of a ferry leaving the harbor for the seven-mile run to Woods Hole. Cynthia and I wordlessly reminisced about our son, overjoyed that he had been given the chance to experience that beautiful island for so many summers and to be embraced there by the incredible people of Camp Jabberwocky. We shed tears from our still-fresh grief. But, even then, some of the tears flowed from the wonder we felt for the singular blessing that Graham had been ours and always would be.

Eventually, our random paddling brought us alongside a sturdy little lobster boat. Remarkably, the name on the light green stern read *Sea Glass*. Happenstance or not, it was clearly my signal to hand over Jamie's discovery to Cynthia. I told her the story and held out the little box from

Beadnik's. As I had been, Graham's mother was stunned by the tiny object and the circumstances of its discovery. We paddled quietly for another hour before pulling Graham's kayak up onto the sand at Owen Park.

Later that summer, I returned to the Vineyard to clear my mind and do some writing about Graham. I took long walks on our special stretch of State Beach, continually looking down at the wet sand under my bare feet. In the exact place where Jamie had found the glass heart, there were countless shells and stones, but, curiously, there was no beach glass there. None at all.

Not a single piece.

"I am struck by the sense that most of us lead a life of disability, the disability of distance and restraint. It is the one disability not in evidence at Camp Jabberwocky."
—Sarah Putnam, *HOPE* magazine

On the first day of camp that summer after Graham's passing, I read, alphabetically, through the health histories that the campers must provide at the beginning of each Jabberwocky session. I wanted to refresh my memory about their medical and social issues. At the end of the thick ring-bound notebook was a file on Sam Wood, a young man with Down Syndrome I had known for a number of years. Perhaps due to his dark beard and linebacker's build, Sam might appear gruff to someone meeting him for the first time. This thoughtful man, however, is as far from gruff as a human being can be. Like many other people with the chromosomal condition called Trisomy 21, Sam's personality is characterized by a profound gentleness and an inherent affection for all kinds of people. We are always very happy to have several campers with Down Syndrome at Jabberwocky.

After reading through Sam's medical forms, I walked down to the Vineyard Haven ferry terminal with the excited, crazily dressed collection of counselors who, by tradition, greet the campers coming off the boat with flamboyant cheers and songs. One of the first campers walking down the gangway, an enormous smile on his face, was another camper named Sam, Sam Stoddard, a much-loved young man with Down Syndrome. He was sporting a T-shirt that said, "I have an extra chromosome and I know how to use it." He was followed closely by Kendra, Michaela, Skye and still another Sam (called "Rhyno" for short, an affectionate contraction of his last name), four more campers with Down Syndrome, uniformly cherished by everyone at Camp. A few moments later, Sam Wood walked carefully down the ramp and was swallowed into the loud collective embrace of Camp Jabberwocky.

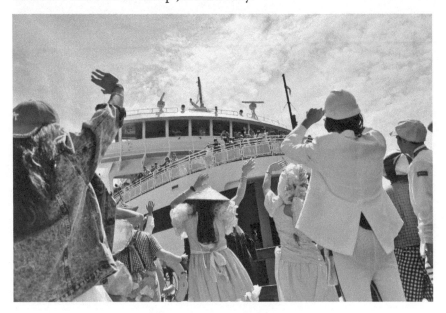

The welcome at the ferry terminal

In the raucous crowd at the ferry terminal, It occurred to me that the three Sams, Kendra, Michaela and Skye indeed know how to use their extra twenty-first chromosomes—they spread kindness and humanity in our world, although I doubt that any genetics researcher could explain that in terms of DNA sequences.

As Sam Wood walked away from the ferry terminal with his counselor, I recalled a section on his health form that made me chuckle: "Loves food and will eat just about anything." I also recalled a section in which a physician had said that "his intellectual disability can cause slow processing time and some difficulty verbally expressing himself."

That afternoon I was sitting on the big swing on the porch of the main cabin by myself, thinking about Graham and all we had experienced together at Jabberwocky. My heart was full, as it often is in that special place.

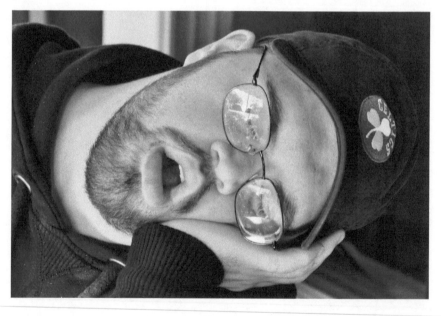

Sam

Sam Wood approached from the direction of his cabin, quietly sat down next to me on the swing and, in a gesture that was completely natural, rested his head gently on my shoulder. In a barely audible voice that was steady and soothing, he said, "I miss Graham. I love Graham. I love you. That will never change."

What a wonderful world it would be, I thought—if we all had such difficulty expressing ourselves.

Cynthia volunteered to do some cooking for camp, allowing Amy, the regular cook, an occasional well-deserved respite. Graham's mom did not mind rising early to give the campers and counselors a special treat, like her thick French toast made from challah bread and topped with fresh berries from the Morning Glory Farm and Vermont maple syrup. Cynthia stayed at her friend Andrea's beautiful home on the harbor in Edgartown, near the ferry to Chappaquiddick. I visited her in that alluring place where land and sea meet, and we watched the little ferryboats shuttling bikes and cars across the narrow channel. Both of us were struggling mightily with the bittersweet experience of Camp at that time, desperately missing our son, while absorbing an abundance of life-giving "Jabberwocky love."

Absentmindedly looking around Andrea's sunny home, I noticed a volume of poetry on a coffee table and picked it up. I opened it, turned randomly to a page in the middle and started reading. It was a verse from a poem by a local poet called *Loss of a Beloved One*, by Henny Darrell:

"*When lights are burning low*
and life has slipped away
when all I love is gone
why should I stay?
When so much love was spent
don't let it be in vain
what seems forever lost
will be eternal gain."

Early on in our camp session that first year without Graham, one experience overwhelmingly confirmed that the decision to go had been the right one. I offered to take some campers out in Vineyard Haven harbor in the inflatable tandem kayak that had meant so much to Graham and me. Paddling around that sun-splashed cove was a new activity for our camp session and, as was the case with golf at Mink Meadows a few years earlier, it was a proud feeling to add a new sport to the growing menu of camp activities. Most of the campers who ventured out had never been in a kayak, and it was thrilling to see them challenging themselves and, above all, having fun. On our kayaking days, small groups of campers and counselors rode the short distance from Camp to the harbor in a couple of vans and my dusty Jeep Grand Cherokee with Graham's initials on its license plates. With pop tunes like "Good Vibrations" blasting out of wide-open windows, we shared the uniquely summery anticipation of heading for the beach on a sunny morning. From a sandy spot next to the town dock, it was easy to launch the kayak into the picturesque harbor bordered by dune grasses and weathered shingled homes.

On the first of those halcyon summer days, I marveled as David (with his counselor Samantha), Elke (with Sarah), Michaela (with Kate) and Skye (with Tina) took turns paddling in one of the island's most beautiful settings, campers in the front of Graham's kayak and their counselors right behind them in "the backseat." It was thrilling to see joy on the faces of old and new camp friends, knowing that Graham's kayak was again serving as a vehicle for adventure.

An amazing person had arrived at Camp for the first time that summer. Patricia Keleher was forty-five years old and lived in a group home in New Hampshire due to cerebral palsy that confined her to a wheelchair and made it difficult for her to speak. But Patty's zest for life was evident the instant we saw her being wheeled down the gangway from the ferry. There were very few moments, in fact, during the next month when there was not an infectious smile beaming on her face, as she experienced the zany culture of Camp Jabberwocky for the first time. Every time I looked at Patty, I was awestruck. Her lean body had been twisted by cerebral palsy, but an aura of pure joy radiated from her face. She literally seemed unable to stop smiling.

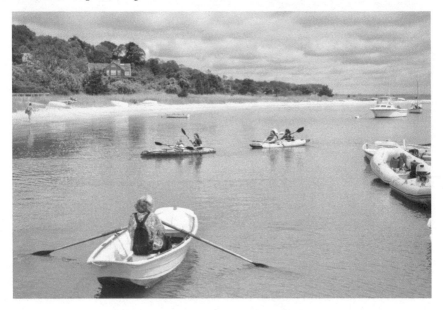

Vineyard Haven Harbor.

Mary Beth Rush—known at Camp as "MB"—a funny and joyous high school student from Sudbury, Massachusetts, had already been at Jabberwocky by then for a couple of years. MB's uniquely sunny attitude and wacky sense of humor were well known to us by then. From her wheelchair, despite athetosis that made coordinated movement difficult, MB led a life packed with fun and achievement. She was an honor student, a disc jockey with her own radio program and a beautiful young woman in every sense of the word.

On a particularly glorious late June day, Patty and MB went kayaking for the first time ever, with their counselors, Meghan and Julia. Patty and MB needed help getting into the kayak and, one at a time, their counselors and I carried them from the beach and slipped them into position.

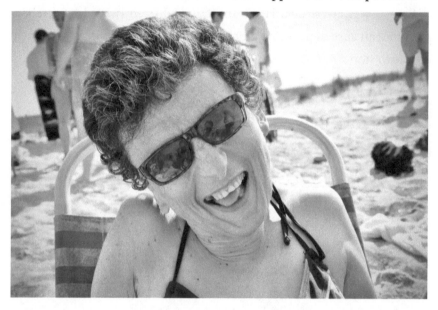

Patty

First, Meghan and I carried Patty out and helped her get comfortable in Graham's front seat. With effortless athleticism from her volleyball career at Colgate, Meghan paddled them out into the harbor, while Patty fiercely gripped her paddle, and I sprinted down the dock to get some photos, glowing with the pride of a parent watching a child ride a bike for the first time. A half-hour later, when Meghan and Patty cruised back in, it was MB's turn. We lifted Patty out, plunked her on a beach towel, and Julia and I carried MB out and settled her into Graham's seat.

As Julia and I were lowering MB into the kayak, Meghan called from the beach and yelled, "Hey, Dr. Steve, Patty says she loves you!"

Before I could even begin to marvel at that statement, MB smiled up at me from Graham's old spot in the front of our kayak and said, " I love you too, Dr. Steve."

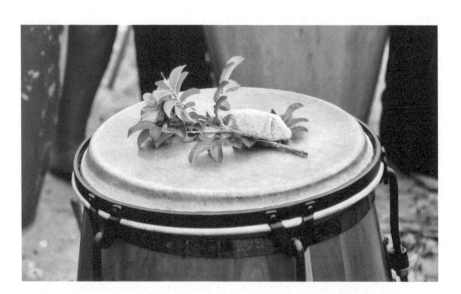

The adjective most often applied to Rick Bausman is *exuberant*. The *Vineyard Gazette* has described the Martha's Vineyard percussionist, teacher and songwriter as a contemporary pied piper, the perfect title for a man who draws all kinds of people into a joyful parade of music and passion for life. With his sandy hair and faded T-shirts, Rick still looks—and sometimes acts—like a kid, even after more than two decades of performing and teaching drumming on Martha's Vineyard to people with and without disabilities. Rick has been a Camp Jabberwocky volunteer forever, and his barefoot, flamboyant presence has been a fixture on the Vineyard for as long as most islanders can remember. Musically, he draws upon a myriad of styles, including traditional percussion rhythms from Haiti and Africa. By creating adaptive devices for the drums and drumsticks, Rick inspires people with physical and mental challenges to create music with him. In the process, he ends up teaching self-esteem, the satisfaction of being part of a community and how to laugh at one another and ourselves.

Rick's work sometimes requires uncanny patience. During a music class at Camp, I watched that calm perseverance as he taught Graham to "play" the conga. By experimenting with a variety of sticks, mallets and brushes attached with Velcro to Graham's hands, Rick gradually coaxed Graham's nervous system to relax, ultimately allowing him to produce some rewarding thwaps on a big Cuban conga.

Rick's group performs periodically at State Beach in the hours leading up to sunset when the weather is warm. The entire Vineyard community is welcome at these celebrations of the season simply referred to as "Drumming at the Beach." Scores of people turn out to listen and dance in the sand alongside Camp Jabberwocky in the golden light at the end of a summer day. When Camp gathered for Drumming at the Beach for the first time in 2010, our initial experience there without Graham, Rick and his group placed a conga in the sand at the very center of the musicians. It sat there unplayed, with a beach rose resting on it.

"This day is your life."

—Jean Jacques Rousseau

At Camp Jabberwocky and its sister camps, life is experienced in the present. The counselors and campers live in the now. Each day is a clean slate to be filled up with fresh experience and laughter. There is very little fretting about yesterday or tomorrow at Jabberwocky. When I volunteer there, I try to adopt that spirit of carpe diem, although it does not necessarily come naturally to me. I watch the campers living in the moment and I try to be more like them. When I'm lingering in a warm outdoor shower at night, looking up at the stars and moon through a canopy of oak leaves, and I've forgotten what day of the week it is, I know that I'm getting closer to their state of mind.

At Andrea's house in Edgartown, I happened on another of Henny Darrell's spare poems called *Lost Chance*:

> *"Everyone is busy with their task*
> *but may I ask:*
> *'Have you noticed this beautiful day?'*
> *'No way we don't have time,'*
> *they say."*

Clearly, the poet was not referring to Camp Jabberwocky. For many of the campers—and volunteers—their time on the island is the capstone of an entire year and they are not about to waste a moment of it.

Each summer I made a point of stopping at Beadniks, the arts and crafts store in Vineyard Haven, to buy token gifts, typically earrings or bracelets for Graham's counselors. It was a vibrant place filled with sunlight, colorful beads, handcrafted jewelry and the aroma of burning incense. Outside, a sign read *Don't Worry Bead Happy*.

During the summer after Graham passed away, an instinct told me to stop at Beadniks again. I wandered the aisles for a few minutes before stumbling on a weathered wooden box filled with small ceramic cubes with letters etched on them. A pleasant young woman named Melanie, who was preparing to study metalsmithing at Bridgewater State College, asked if I needed help. After we brainstormed for a few minutes, she volunteered to create thirteen bracelets, each a different color, using cubes engraved with Graham's alliterative initials. The bracelets would be tokens of gratitude for the wonderful people who had cared for him so passionately during his thirteen summers on the island.

Buying presents for Graham's counselors was peculiar in a way because, like all the volunteers at Camp, they expected nothing in return for their efforts. They unpretentiously embodied Emerson's notion that "the only true gift is a portion of thyself." The one reward they hoped for was to see their campers smiling and laughing. Fully understanding that, my hope was that wearing the whimsical bracelets would remind Graham's counselors that what they gave him will never be lost and that a portion of Graham remains in each of them.

Walking up to Beadniks to collect the finished bracelets a few days later, I found myself smiling at a vivid memory from exactly a year earlier, Graham's last summer at Camp. It was a vignette that perfectly epitomized the experiences he shared with his counselors over the years. The incident occurred on our last day on the island, during a sudden torrential downpour, the kind that causes flash flooding.

I was driving up Main Street in Vineyard Haven, past the ice cream shops and ancient movie theater, windshield wipers oscillating furiously, when I happened upon Jackie and Kaitlin, Graham's counselors at the time, frantically wheeling him in the direction of Camp. They had been caught in the sudden cloudburst. Jackie and Kaitlin had removed their jackets and were holding them like a tent over Graham while they were pelted by enormous drops of rain falling almost as violently as hail. I pulled alongside the threesome and, through a wall of water, asked if they wanted to get in the Jeep with me and ride back to Camp.

"No thanks, Dr. Steve, we're just fine!" shouted Kaitlin.

As they ran up Main Street in the direction of Camp, the two counselors pushing frantically on either side of Graham's wheelchair, drenched as thoroughly as if they had jumped in the harbor, Jackie, Kaitlin and Graham were—naturally—howling with laughter.

"There is a sacredness in tears. They speak more eloquently than ten thousand tongues. They are the messengers of grief ... of unspeakable love."
—Washington Irving

Those of us who have spent time at Camp Jabberwocky and Zeno Mountain Farm are honored to have a friend named Paul Remy. When he appears at Camp each summer, I watch him with ever-growing amazement.

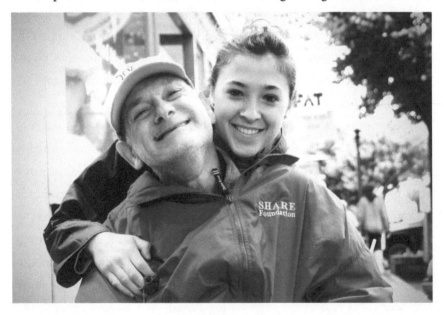

Paul with Christina

Paul came to Camp sixty years ago as a youngster in a cumbersome wheelchair, newly diagnosed with cerebral palsy. Along with a handful of campers from the early days, Paul became a pioneer in showing what people with disabilities can accomplish and how much fun can be had while accomplishing it. While his CP prevents him from walking or performing routine tasks without assistance, Paul's mind is keen and his spirit unshakable. He has a profoundly compassionate heart and never seems bitter. He is a skilled writer who contributes articles to the *Vineyard Gazette* and other newspapers, examining the role of people with disabilities in society with honesty and humor. His writing is done painstakingly by working a keyboard with adaptive tools that he helped design.

Paul has thinning gray hair now and a face wrinkled with laugh lines—well-earned during decades of silliness at Jabberwocky and Zeno. It amazes me to think that his broad, silly grin has been a fixture at the camps for more than half a century. Graham's CP physically resembled Paul's. They had similar issues with spasticity and trouble controlling their muscles. But, over time, Paul learned to communicate quite eloquently despite those challenges. I always asked for his thoughts on what might help Graham express himself more effectively, but, for some reason, we never found a tool that was very helpful.

The emotions that filled me during the first camp session without Graham in 2010 were sometimes overwhelming. Grief lurked in many familiar places where I had spent time joyfully with my son. At the same time, my heart was gladdened by the environment of love that abounds at Camp. From time to time, I found deserted places where I could cry— tears seemingly flowing from both emotions at the same time. But even though, in private, I let my feelings out periodically, there remained a well of emotion inside me. I held it in as long as I could, until one rainy day toward the end of my time on the island. As I walked through the main cabin, I spotted Paul at a table by himself. He was working on his laptop with a prong-like gadget attached to his forehead that he used to hit the keys.

I stopped in my tracks, transfixed by the sight of that graceful man and his noble spirit. The miracle of Camp Jabberwocky, my love for Graham, my terrible sense of loss, my gratitude for Graham's life—all of it—suddenly felt like a dam ready to burst. Turning his neck very slightly, Paul looked at me and I saw that he *understood*. I ran to him, grabbed him from behind in a bear hug and wept a small waterfall of tears onto his neck and the headrest of his wheelchair. Although he had not actually moved, I had an unmistakable feeling that Paul had grabbed me and wrapped me in the "Jabberwocky love" that I needed so desperately in those moments.

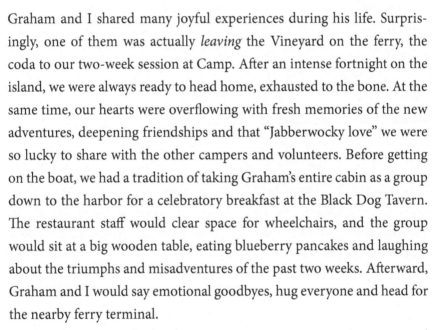

Graham and I shared many joyful experiences during his life. Surprisingly, one of them was actually *leaving* the Vineyard on the ferry, the coda to our two-week session at Camp. After an intense fortnight on the island, we were always ready to head home, exhausted to the bone. At the same time, our hearts were overflowing with fresh memories of the new adventures, deepening friendships and that "Jabberwocky love" we were so lucky to share with the other campers and volunteers. Before getting on the boat, we had a tradition of taking Graham's entire cabin as a group down to the harbor for a celebratory breakfast at the Black Dog Tavern. The restaurant staff would clear space for wheelchairs, and the group would sit at a big wooden table, eating blueberry pancakes and laughing about the triumphs and misadventures of the past two weeks. Afterward, Graham and I would say emotional goodbyes, hug everyone and head for the nearby ferry terminal.

As I drove onto the big boat sitting next to my son, I experienced something very close to perfect contentment. Graham filled me with happiness. He was so gentle, so resilient—so *good*. He was a wondrous companion and, of all the men on the earth, he needed *me*.

And I needed *him* just as much, or, perhaps, a little more.

In addition, the trillions of cells in Graham's body contained the DNA of Cynthia's and my ancestors. Traces of my mother and father, my grandparents, my brother, my aunts and my cousins, all those other people I have loved, were in his chromosomes, in the set of his jaw and in his high cheekbones. Sitting side by side in the Jeep, departing that beautiful island, Graham and I were part of a continuum on the earth. In fact, as we took our leave of the Vineyard, we were really members now of *two* families—our biological relatives *and* the extended family of Camp Jabberwocky, the mosaic progeny of Helen Lamb.

However, inconceivably, after thirteen summers together on the island, Graham was no longer beside me in 2010 as I left Vineyard Haven on a boat called Katama. I tried to take some comfort from having been there with Graham for all those years—to persuade myself that we had had a pretty good run. But not being able to rub my hand on the back of his silky head next to me in the passenger seat was an exquisite agony. I made no effort to hide my tears from the other passengers as I watched the island slowly recede in the churning water of the big ferry's wake. In those moments on the boat and long after the Jeep crossed the Cape Cod Canal and joined the frenetic aggression of the traffic on Route 3 north, my whole being ached. Yet, even in that state of anguish, I was acutely aware of an epiphany that had been slowly crystallizing during those halcyon summers on Martha's Vineyard—Graham opened the door to a world in which love is all that matters.

15

GODFATHER

Cynthia and I could never stop kissing Graham. Throughout his entire life, even after he became a strapping young man, it was just a natural thing for us to do, and we did it unabashedly nearly every moment we were with him. We wanted Graham to know, millisecond by millisecond, how much he was loved. At the same time, those tender gestures made his parents feel full and happy. Lisa, his dear friend from Crotched Mountain, let us know that Graham was amused by the apparent competition between his parents to see who could hug him the most.

Inescapably, Graham's days started with effusive gestures of endearment, wherever he was. Regardless of the weather, Cynthia loved to wake him up by singing the wonderfully hokey theme song from *Mr. Roger's Neighborhood*:

> *"It's a beautiful day in the neighborhood*
> *A neighborly way in the beauty wood*
> *Won't you be mine*
> *Won't you be mine?"*

Graham would respond to this corny musical alarm with a pained look, before giving his mom a wry smile to greet the new day.

I took a memorable photo of Graham on a trip to Bermuda in which he appears to be puckering up for a kiss. Cynthia asked for a print of it and, after Graham died, she took the picture everywhere and kissed it whenever she was thinking of him—which was most of the time. A short while after Graham's passing, Cynthia was in Manhattan making an effort to get back to work, primarily for the sake of distraction. Climbing out of a cab on Fifth Avenue on a particularly nasty late winter morning, she made eye contact with a curious stranger approaching her on the crosswalk. Emerging from a veil of sleet, he looked to her like a character from *Oliver Twist,* a shadowy, waif-like presence, somehow not of this world. The pedestrians on the crosswalk were bent against the elements, gazing at the pavement and hurrying forward. The gaunt figure before Cynthia, however, suddenly stopped and looked into her eyes. She had the impression that he had materialized from another place and time.

With a kind expression, he asked, "Isn't it a beautiful day?"

She was taken aback, but managed to reply, "Yes—I guess it depends on how you look at it."

"Enjoy this beautiful day," he said, before disappearing in the crush of commuters dashing down the sidewalk in the mist.

Cynthia ducked into a coffee shop to escape the freezing rain. Over the bustle of the cafe, she became aware of the iconic Motown sound of the Four Tops on ceiling speakers. As she took her place in line, her entire being quivering with raw emotion, she recognized a familiar verse and refrain:

> *"In and out of my life*
> *You come and you go*
> *Leaving just your picture behind*

And I've kissed it a thousand times
Sugar Pie Honey Bunch
You know that I love you."

Graham and I had treasured our kayaking and swimming at Sunset Lake at the base of Crotched Mountain. The warm days of summer are fleeting in the White Mountains, and we savored them during the occasional weekends we spent together at the school. It was on Sunset Lake that we discovered how well-suited we were for kayaking, using the two-person inflatable canoe that was comfortable and safe. Moving on the smooth water was soothing for us both. In that placid haven, bordered by solemn pine trees, we experienced a sense of freedom from physical forces that normally constrained us. To honor the years that Graham spent at Crotched and to celebrate the happy memories we had of the lake, Cynthia and I decided to scatter some of Graham's ashes in that special body of water. We packed a picnic and the kayak and arranged to meet Lisa, who was still working at the school.

We sat in beach chairs for a while, catching up with Graham's friend at our familiar spot on the waterfront. When the time felt right, Cynthia and I inflated the kayak and paddled out from the sandy beach, carrying the surreal plastic container that held Graham's ashes. In the middle of the lake, we turned and faced the mountain. The school campus and Graham's old dorm were hidden from view, high up in the forest with its lofty canopy of white birch and fir trees that rose above a spongy floor of ferns, moss and wildflowers. The sun shimmered on the lake's clear spring water on a perfect summer day.

Cynthia and I spoke to Graham for a few moments and, in what felt like a dream, took turns pouring the haunting gray granules into the lake. Graham's ashes, illuminated from above, formed a glistening green cloud in the water around the kayak. A moment later, the sun broke free of a lone cumulous cloud and shone brilliantly. Beams of light bent under the water in golden columns that sparkled with the sinking ashes. It was bizarre and heart-rending to think that the particles creating that fantastic play of light and shadow had once formed the tissues of the beautiful human being we loved so much.

Cynthia and I paddled quietly for a while longer, watching the poignant visual effect slowly fade until it disappeared with the current toward the base of Crotched Mountain.

For a long time, I wondered what to do with Graham's clothing. There were nearby drop boxes for Goodwill and the Salvation Army, but I was looking for something else; I just didn't know what. On a midwinter day, I drove to Chelsea, a vibrant, densely populated city of immigrants separated from Boston by the Mystic River. I was working on a photo essay about MGH's community health centers, facilities that serve working-class neighborhoods around Boston. The Chelsea Healthcare Center provides desperately needed medical and social services in ten languages to adults and children from countless backgrounds. Many of the clinic's patients are refugees fleeing civil war, violence and persecution in homelands far away.

That morning, I took a walk with my camera through a hardscrabble neighborhood lined with triple-decker row houses. Many of the tenements had fallen into disrepair, but on the faces of families rushing in and out of doorways, there were looks of optimism that, for some reason, I hadn't expected. I walked a few more blocks before the significance of those hopeful expressions sunk in—in that outwardly inauspicious place, America's hallowed promise of freedom and opportunity was very much alive. I met a remarkable family from Rwanda that day, thanks to a social worker at the MGH clinic who was assisting them with the mind-boggling transition from rural Africa to inner-city America. She asked if I wanted to join her for a "home visit," to see how they were doing in an apartment she had found for them, and I eagerly accepted.

They were a loving, happy family, cruelly displaced, yet seemingly unbroken. They needed absolutely everything to start over again. It was the MGH social worker's job to serve as their guide and advocate. The family had survived genocide and traumatic years in refugee camps. I knew I would never really comprehend what had happened to them. Sitting with them in their spartan apartment, I marveled at their capacity to smile and even laugh with us. There were four lovely girls and a boy about twelve years old. The lad seemed self-confident and made steady eye contact. He watched me closely with a beaming, gap-toothed smile. I noted that he was about Graham's size. His name was Fabrice. No thought was required. I knew then what Graham would want me to do with his winter clothes.

Conversing with them haltingly, as my colleague translated from Kinyarwanda, a language I didn't know existed, I felt Graham's presence. I sensed that he wanted to lend his solidarity to this family that had endured the unimaginable and now needed help. I thought it would be unseemly to talk about my personal loss at that time and, possibly, rude to broach the subject of giving my son's winter garments to the boy. So, I dropped them off at the clinic a few days later for the staff to deliver to Fabrice anonymously. The image of that friendly boy from central Africa wearing Graham's ski parka made me smile. Fabrice's new jacket would be a tangible link between two young men who should have had no worldly connection. I wondered about that on the ride home.

Increasingly, I was developing a conviction that, in Rabbi Lawrence Kushner's words, there were "invisible lines of connection" among people in the world. In a literal sense, the clothing that Graham could no longer use would protect a boy fleeing one of the most dangerous places in the world against the bitter cold of winter in New England. But an instinct told me something more might be going on. Walking into my home and passing through Graham's room, I wondered if there was now a connection between my son and Fabrice that was beyond my understanding.

Sneakers are, admittedly, odd things to collect. Yet, for almost twenty-three years, I saved every pair that Graham wore. There was something sentimental about marking the passage of time with that collection of ever-enlarging shoes. Some families measure the growing heights of children over time with pencil marks on closet doors. For me, it was the sneakers. For a while, I lined them up on the right side of a stairway that leads to the second floor, the smallest pair on the bottom step, the largest on top. When all the steps were occupied, sneakers started making their way down the other side, getting ever bigger as they descended. Eventually, a day came when it was hazardous to walk up or down the stairway.

I decided to move the sneakers to a guest room, where the collection sat in a disorderly pile. Somewhere in the mound was a pair of white leather baby shoes with a price tag still attached to the sole. Like all the others, they had been carefully chosen by Graham's mom. Because he was never really able to walk, none of the shoes had much wear. Most of them were rubber and canvas high tops with only minor blemishes. Surprisingly, when I looked at specific pairs, even some of the oldest ones, I could recall corresponding times in Graham's life. I loved every one of those sneakers simply because they were his. I also sensed that one day I would find a purpose for that singular collection of shoes.

The answer came to me when I was given the opportunity to work in Haiti. When I accepted the assignment, I pictured taking the entire sneaker collection and giving it away at a camp in Port-au-Prince. But air travel to Haiti was still in a state of chaos. I hadn't considered the uncertainty of checking the sizable collection of shoes, occupying several duffel bags, on a flight to a place in a condition very close to anarchy. Recent travelers to Haiti suggested that I would probably never see the sneakers again if I did.

So, instead, I decided to take a single pair of the sneakers with me in my carry-on luggage as a symbol. I knew that I would surely meet a kid about the right age who would be grateful to have them. Giving away even that one pair of sneakers would mean that a palpable remnant of Graham's goodness had been given to the people of Haiti, a rubber and canvas symbol of solidarity with people facing adversity. On my first night in Port-au-Prince, sweating on a cot under a tangled mosquito net, I had a vivid dream. Graham had taken on the frail body of a Haitian boy. He was able to walk. I watched him emerge from a dark alley into a crumbling street and disappear into the night. I woke up and, for a few panicky moments, had no idea where I was. I struggled to fall back to sleep in the stifling heat, filled with apprehension about what lay ahead.

In the morning, I climbed into a dusty van crammed with volunteers from several countries. There was nervous chatter in French, Creole and English as we passed the rubble of what was left of entire neighborhoods. The vehicle labored and lurched on rutted dirt roads until we entered a surreal landscape. We had arrived at the tent city of Delmas, where some 50,000 survivors of the earthquake were living in unimaginable squalor. A sprawling tent there housed our makeshift medical clinic. A drove of small pigs was foraging in mud just outside the entrance. The Delmas tent city—and our clinic—had arisen on a massive toxic waste site, the only open land in Port-au-Prince where people had been able to flee during the earthquake. The air was a putrid miasma of vapors from nearby latrines and festering garbage.

Near the entrance to the camp, I was shocked to see a group of boys playing soccer. The "field" they were playing on was nothing more than a flattened area in a massive rubbish dump, bordered by a huge cement drainage ditch littered with refuse. Each morning we passed the field in our van. The boys were always there. Graham's pair of sneakers was in my backpack with granola bars, a few valuables and some medical supplies.

I took a break from the clinic one sweltering afternoon and walked over to the field. A young father was watching his son playing soccer in that heartbreaking place. The boy was barefoot. The moment had come to give away Graham's sneakers.

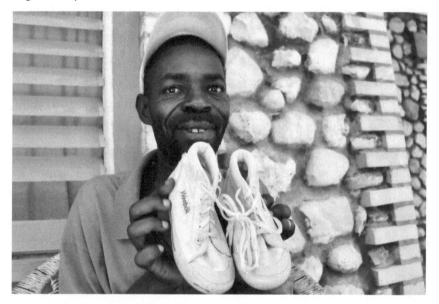

The idea that Kate Farrell and Graham Gardner were married in another life was absolutely believable. In fact, when Kate visited a medium in New Hampshire, the woman told her that she and Graham had been man and wife in another lifetime in England and that Graham had made wheels for carts. Cartwheels!

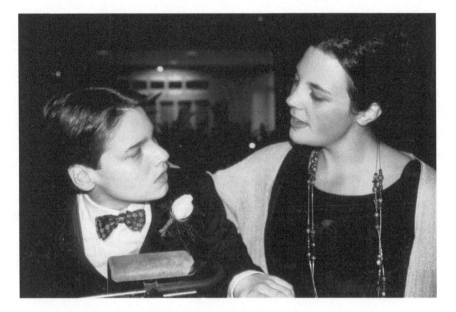

Graham and Kate

They were very happy together, said the medium, and Graham was "an advanced spiritual being filled with a radiant light." Kate already knew this last part was true. She and Graham had a bond so spiritual that it was impossible to imagine that it had not been forged over a long period of time. A longer time, it seemed to Cynthia and me, than Graham had been with us in this life. Kate called Graham "a brother, a son, a friend and a teacher."

This luminous young woman was oblivious to her own natural beauty, but Graham loved to gaze at her sparkling green eyes, chestnut hair and porcelain skin. Kate was twenty-one when she started helping us with Graham, while he was still just a youngster of eleven or twelve. It was a period characterized by both challenges and triumphs. There were alarming stretches when Graham was in constant distress, including the weeks following his harrowing stay at Children's Hospital. During that time, Cynthia and I sometimes fought bitterly over what was best for our son. On some of those occasions, it was Kate's calming presence that got us through, one day at a time.

An innate understanding existed between Graham and Kate, a communication that sometimes seemed otherworldly. Even though Graham could not form words, Kate knew exactly what he was feeling from moment to moment. When Kate gave Graham a bath and groomed him for bed, his room became a magical spa warmed by candlelight and transformed by incense and fantastic stories. There was an aura of tenderness and love in the room that existed nowhere else. Kate shared this, her "most profound memory" of Graham:

> "One night, I was feeding him dinner. I'm not sure what we had been discussing, but I said, 'You're the Buddha incarnate, aren't you?' and Graham burst out laughing! He was absolutely howling with laughter (you remember how he would do that!). And then he stopped, leaned forward and looked me straight in the eye, his eyes all twinkling, as in, 'You got me!' And I started to cry. Not tears of sadness, but tears of utter admiration and appreciation because I was in the presence of pure greatness. I still get goosebumps when I think about that moment.
>
> The Buddha is an enlightened being who comes to Earth to teach us about compassion. He teaches us to live in the moment, to love and to laugh. This was Graham's message. Rather, I should say, this is Graham's message, as it continues to be so."

Kate became a massage therapist before, unsurprisingly, choosing a career working with people with disabilities at a day program. She now has a husband and a son of her own. She discovered she was pregnant one week before Graham died. "What if?" she wondered.

When I returned from Haiti, there was the question of what to do with Graham's remaining sneakers. The answer became clear when I met a little boy named Quinn and learned that he was Graham's godson. Yes— Graham was a godfather!

Cynthia and I agreed that Kate Farrell's baby boy— Graham's godson— should inherit the sneakers, with the fervent hope that he would wear out every pair, walking the earth with a joyful heart and running on it with abandon.

With her permission, here are some excerpts from Kate Farrell's note to me about the decision she made with her husband, Chris, to posthumously make Graham the godfather of their son Quinn:

"I found out that I was pregnant on January 31, 2010. One week later, Graham passed away. I was stunned when my mother gave me the news. How could that be? I had not seen Graham in person in eight years. I couldn't accept the fact that I never would again. The regret of allowing those years to slip by without seeing Graham jabs at my heart.

Before the initial shock had even worn off, the next thought I had was of the new life growing inside me. I couldn't help but think that maybe Graham's spirit is coming back to Earth, this time as my child. I still wonder about it sometimes when I am watching Quinn, but my instinct tells me that he is not Graham.

As I've written to you before, I think Graham was an enlightened being. Enlightened beings choose to come to Earth to restore dharma (at its essence, the embodiment of just and decent behavior) in times of great imbalance. They bless us with their teachings and their lessons go on long after their physical manifestations depart. I believe that Graham's soul does not need to reincarnate to settle karmic debts like the rest of us. He was perfect! He never hurt anyone. He was never selfish, unkind or greedy. He was completely pure of heart.

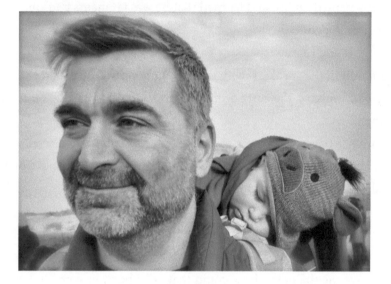

Quinn and his dad

Now that he is gone, we are seeing what a tremendous impact he made on Earth. And the ripple effect continues. Brahman is a central concept in Hinduism. It signifies the ultimate reality. I try to mindfully practice grasping this concept every day. The way I understand it is to accept that God is everything we see and everything we don't see; that God lives inside each one of us and we dwell fully in God; that there is nothing outside of God and that God is love. I truly believe that Graham got that, every second of every minute that he was here with us, and he hasn't really left us at all.

So, with the guidance of Graham's indelible spirit and through the stories we will share of his exemplary life, may my son, Quinn, attain a true understanding of God.

Isn't that the whole point of being a godparent?"

Most of us have experienced the eerie feeling that goes with handling the personal possessions of a loved one who has passed away. Ordinary objects take on surprising poignancy. Everyday items are suddenly heirlooms to be handed down and treasured. Cynthia and I knew we were carrying this sentimentalism to the extreme, but many of the things that Graham left behind became nothing short of sacred to us. Sorting through Graham's drawers, for example, I experienced a melodramatic twinge while staring at his hairbrush! The little wooden stick with its crooked bristles was sacred because it had groomed his satiny hair. I came very close to weeping at the sight of his deodorant stick! A crinkled tube of Tom's Silly Strawberry toothpaste and his Royal Mandarin cologne were precious artifacts, probably because the scents from those toiletries evoked *Graham* in the deepest parts of my brain.

Clothes, we discovered, were uniquely sacred because they had physically enveloped the person we adored. Graham's soft winter scarf, the down ski jacket that was handed down to Fabrice, the tassel loafers he sported on special occasions, the Teva sandals he wore on trips to the Caribbean are all sacred now. His *Life is Good* T-shirts were particularly touching because they had fit his torso—and his message of hope—so perfectly.

And, of course, there were the sneakers. There was pathos in the sneakers because Graham stood proudly in them when assisted by a parent or friend, but the soles never had the chance to become worn down by walking or running.

It was unfathomable that Graham's familiar belongings were sitting dispassionately in drawers and closets, waiting for the right moment to be given away when the beautiful person who wore them was gone. But, the summer after Graham's passing, it thrilled me to see our matching yellow life jackets back in use, worn by Jabberwocky campers and counselors, paddling and laughing in the Vineyard Haven harbor.

At home, Graham's wheelchair occupied its old spot in the dining room for many months, heartbreakingly empty. The chair became a nearly holy object—the ultimate symbol of a life lived with incomprehensible dignity. It took a long time before I was ready to let it go and donate it to Crotched Mountain.

Searching for something to eat one morning, I discovered that even a frozen container of French toast lovingly prepared long ago by his mom—now encased in a growing shell of permafrost in my freezer—was sacred. It was Graham's favorite breakfast.

Time has passed, but, even now, we part with our son's remaining possessions unhurriedly. It felt wonderful, quite recently, to donate Graham's cushiony sheepskin mattress pad to a friend with cancer who had become bedridden. But I plan to keep the turquoise necklace that I gave him many years ago as a symbol of healing. At least for now.

I flew to Bermuda after Graham's passing to write some of these stories, choosing to stay in the same hotel where he and I had spent that singularly joyful week together. For the first time, I was struck by the elegant features of a vintage Otis elevator car that we had ridden daily during our time there—an ornate chandelier, polished brass handrails and inlaid marble on the floor. One morning I asked the elevator out loud if it knew how lucky it was to have once held the most special of all people within its mahogany walls.

That classic Otis elevator car is a sacred thing.

I was not convinced that Graham was "in a better place," as people often suggest in an effort to provide comfort to loved ones after someone dies. First of all, the scientist in me was skeptical about the logistics of such a place. God would have to have a *really* big room to accommodate billions of good people. And existentially, I kept thinking that Graham should still be here with us. Isn't *this* world a pretty happy place for someone loved abundantly and passionately?

As February 6 approached, impossibly nearing a year after Graham's passing, I felt a creeping apprehension. The winter days were bleak and fleeting. The outside world was frigid and dark. Snow and ice encased the house—and my soul—like a shroud. The beautiful person who had been the nucleus of our universe was simply gone. The guiding light in our world had gone out. The worst possible thing that can happen to a parent had actually happened—to Cynthia and me.

On the eve of that awful anniversary, a card arrived from Donna Chadwick, Graham's beloved music teacher. I waited to open it until the morning when it was exactly one year since we left for our swim at the YMCA. Donna, like Kate Farrell, considered Graham to be a "spiritual master," and I knew that her thoughts would be discerning and soothing. She knew about our family's mystical connection with mourning doves and the cover of her card was blank except for a photograph of two young doves. The message inside was stunning:

"Dear Steven,
I know it is the weekend. Brace your tender heart for the
pain spiking to the surface again. Let it happen.
Doves for you—mourning doves.
With compassionate love for you on the anniversary
of Graham's ascension."
Donna

Ascension! Ascension! I actually smiled and said the word aloud a few times. I liked the way it sounded. I liked the image it evoked. And

I desperately wanted to share Donna's faith. Maybe Graham's work on earth *was* done. Maybe he did need to be freed from his beautiful, but flawed body. Maybe he had returned to God. Maybe he was there—

Among the other angels.

16

STRAIGHT ANGEL

Rosa, a perky seamstress in Salem, whose gentle son, Andrew, passed away as a teenager in a car accident, believes that there are mysterious reasons behind even the most hideous of tragedies. In fact, in Rosa's theology, it was not actually an "accident" that took her son's life that day. Only God has the explanation. She tried to comfort me with that notion after Graham died. Rosa also believes that people like Graham actually choose to come here with disabilities, for reasons that may be impossible for us to understand. Perhaps they come to inspire love in the world.

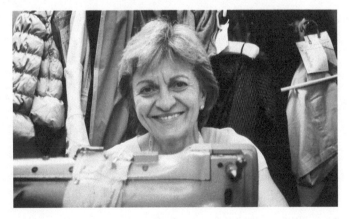

Rosa

I asked her if she would mind explaining her faith in more detail and we talked for a long time in the back of her modest shop, over the pleasant whirring of sewing machines. In crisp English mixed wonderfully with residual syntax from her native Greece, this lovely woman with sparkling dark brown eyes said, "Most people must come down to earth several times for work on their spirit before God accepts them in heaven. Your son, Graham, though, he doesn't need coming back. That boy was straight angel."

"Let the celebration of all our children
And their endless youth
When the world was to them still without problem
Always be that unforgotten Vineyard summer
An everlasting day."
　　　　　—Tomas Napolean, Edgartown poet

At the mouth of Edgartown Harbor, on a crescent-shaped sand bar, a spit of land created by the Great New England Hurricane of 1938, a simple white lighthouse stands proudly above shallow, wind-swept dunes. Feathery beach grasses, outwardly delicate but rooted with enormous strength, bind those dunes against the shifting sands of the tiny peninsula that faces Chappaquiddick Island, just a few hundred yards across the harbor. The Edgartown Lighthouse sits serenely in that place, at the confluence of winding sandy paths bordered by wild New England beach roses that display their vibrant pink blossoms each summer. Around the foundation of that lighthouse is a memorial made of granite cobblestones containing the names of children whose lives were cut short by untimely deaths.

On one of those stones is the name *Graham Hale Gardner.* Rick Harrington, a lifelong Vineyard resident and father of one of the children remembered there, conceived of the memorial and nurtured it into being. The steward of the landmark today is the Martha's Vineyard Museum, while the lighthouse itself, with its flashing red beacon, remains an active aid to navigation of the US Coast Guard. A plaque facing the harbor inlet states:

> *The Children's Lighthouse Memorial*
> *was created with the fervent hope that for the*
> *families of these children, whose interrupted lives*
> *are here remembered, that this lighthouse*
> *be a beacon through the darkness of grief,*
> *reminding and assuring us all with its brightness*
> *that a safe harbor has indeed been reached.*

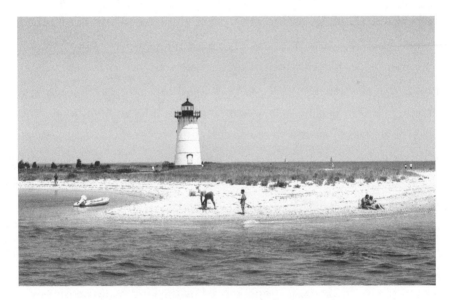

Edgartown Lighthouse

It was Cynthia who discovered this singular place of remembrance and arranged Graham's inclusion in it. His marker was Cynthia's surprise Christmas gift to me at the end of our first year without him. A kindly stonemason named Dudley Levick had set the piece of granite with Graham's name on it in the ground there, on the magical island that had meant so much to all three of us. Cynthia spotted Dudley working there shortly after she arrived on the island in the summer of 2010, his soft blue eyes sparkling behind rimmed glasses, sweating from the effort of his task. Ruddy-faced beneath a tattered straw hat, he was kneeling at the center of a pile of cobblestones, meticulously setting the last pieces of the memorial in place.

Cynthia watched him place a granite marker in the sandy ground with reverence. She bent down to thank him and to share with him some photos of our son so that Dudley could picture the boy whose stone—and memory—he had handled with such care. A few days later, on a sparkling early summer morning, while I was across the island at Camp Jabberwocky, Cynthia walked out to the lighthouse to visit the finished memorial for the first time, acutely aware that she was approaching a hallowed place. She was met in the arched doorway of the lighthouse tower by a slender man with coffee-colored skin. He was smiling and greeting visitors as if he were welcoming them into his own home. The celestial sounds of an aria were reverberating within the conical belly of the lighthouse.

Wade Johnson introduced himself and said he was the keeper of the lighthouse. He added that he was also an overseer of the memorial and, as such, a caretaker for the spirits of the children remembered there. Cynthia stepped back, absorbing that comment, and watched Wade for several minutes as he carefully explained the history of the memorial to groups of visitors. She was deeply moved by the kind man and his obvious devotion to the responsibility he had been given. A few days later, Cynthia and I walked to the lighthouse together on a sandy path from North Water Street. It was my first visit to the memorial, and I could feel my emotions rising. As we neared the structure, my senses became aware of something serene. It took me a moment to realize that it was the music coming from inside the forty-five-foot-high cast-iron tower.

I spotted Wade inside the door and wondered if Mahatma Gandhi had come back to life! The slim, graceful man was wearing a broad smile and a T-shirt that depicted the island's five lighthouses. He gave me a welcome that felt like the embrace of an old friend and walked me over to Graham's stone, where Cynthia was spreading wild rose petals. It was breathtaking to see Graham's name etched in the granite marker. Wade stood with us quietly. I had the curious feeling that he had something to share about Graham. He looked straight into my eyes and said, "Graham's mission was complete."

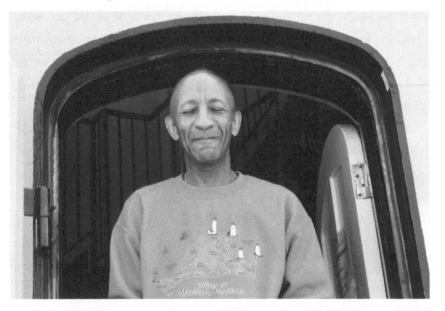

Wade

It was a warm, cloudless morning and Cynthia and I felt lucky to spend some time with the thoughtful man. It was a relatively quiet day, with only a few tourists requiring his attention. Wade explained his conviction about Graham to us and said that the spirits of all the memorialized children were present right there, where land and sea meet in unbroken harmony. As I listened, I began to sense that there was a double meaning to Wade's title of "light keeper." While he monitored the structure of the lighthouse and its beacon, it was equally clear that Wade intended to do his part to keep alive the light that Graham and the other children shone on this world. The Children's Memorial was conceived, in fact, as a place where that light will never fade.

Cynthia and I learned a little about Wade's eclectic past that morning. Before studying at Williams and Vassar, he had operated an ice cream truck. *Perfect*, I thought! A job that brought joy to children. I teased him about being the "good humor man," but I wasn't really joking. Within five minutes of meeting Wade, I had no doubt that he was a human being whose life work was spreading good humor. His job at the lighthouse was clearly more ministry than management. Cynthia and I were so taken by Wade that we wanted all of Camp to come and meet him, and he kindly agreed.

A few days later, Camp Jabberwocky arrived en masse, pushing and pulling wheelchairs laboriously, but excitedly, down one of the sandy paths. Wade welcomed everyone in his characteristically unhurried fashion and explained the history and mission of the memorial. Then he answered questions, with all of Camp fanned out in a half-circle around him in the sand at the base of the lighthouse.

At that moment, I was standing on the circular outside walk of the lantern room, at the top of the lighthouse tower, looking straight down at Wade as he addressed Camp Jabberwocky. The campers and counselors clustered around Wade were people whose lives were marked by kindness, resilience and joy. They had loved Graham and always will.

I was spellbound.

In response to a question from a camper about the memorial, I heard Wade say:

"The souls of these children are always communicating.
Some of us can hear them and some cannot.
The souls here at the base of the lighthouse
are spiritual donors sending energy to those
who go to the top and look out onto the world.
There is a healing in that for us all.
The light that shines here is a celebration of life."

I felt an aura around the lighthouse in those moments that recalled the feelings we experienced in Old North Church at the celebration of Graham's life. From my perch, I gazed past the northeast side of the memorial where Graham's stone lay and into the blue vastness of Nantucket Sound stretching to the horizon. I was profoundly aware that I was experiencing indelible moments of grace that I would carry for the rest of my life. When Wade finished speaking, everyone from camp wanted to climb the spiral stairs inside the lighthouse. But visitors must ascend the last ten feet on a vertical ladder to reach the breathtaking circular platform or "gallery" at the top, where I was standing. I doubted that any visitor in a wheelchair had ever made it up that vertical ladder and all the way to the platform in the history of the lighthouse.

But, needless to say, it never even occurred to the Jabberwocky counselors that they couldn't or shouldn't assist campers in wheelchairs all the way up that ladder and out onto the glorious circular landing with its stunning panorama of the harbor and the village of Edgartown. For the next half hour, I marveled as the counselors carefully hoisted campers up the vertical wall and out to that rarified place. In time, the group descended, made its way to the side of the lighthouse and found Graham's stone. The campers and counselors paused there and quietly remembered him in their own ways for a little while.

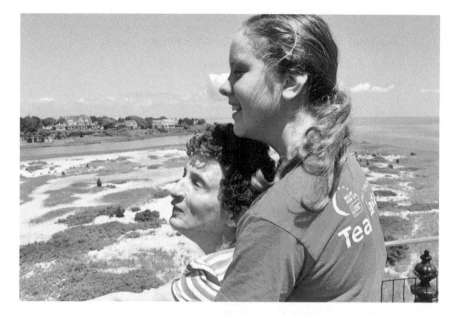

Patty on the gallery with Sarah

Cynthia and I did not want the outing to end mournfully. A picnic had been packed. All we had to do was walk another thirty yards or so past the memorial and we were ready for a day at the beach, with the added bonus of watching a parade of magnificent boats under full sail entering and leaving the harbor. Later, as the counselors pulled their campers back to town along one of the sandy paths, I spotted Wade smiling from the doorway of the lighthouse. In that instant, the world seemed without problem. An unforgettable moment in a Vineyard summer.

An everlasting day.

One of the most robust and vivacious patients in my medical practice at MGH was a lovely octogenarian from Cape Cod named Arlene McCullagh. The white-haired grandmother looked twenty years younger than her age and drove herself up to Boston for annual check-ups. Thankfully, during the time I took care of her, those routine exams never identified any serious medical issues. After her brief exam, I would order some routine tests, we would chat cordially for a few minutes and she was off to beat the traffic to her rustic home on the Cape. Over the years, a friendly relationship developed between us. But, because of her excellent health and the time pressures of modern medicine, I never took the time to learn much about Arlene's personal life. I knew that she was a college graduate and mother of four, having lost a fifth child at birth. I was vaguely aware that she was familiar with Graham's passing and that she had seen his obituary in the Boston Globe. I could sense that she was a spiritual woman and always felt apologetic that our time together was so limited.

At her annual visit, five years after Graham's passing, I asked her about her health and whether any concerns had come up since we last saw one another.

"I've been great, overall. Well, there actually was one scary incident."

"Tell me about it."

"I choked on some food at a restaurant."

"That sounds frightening. What happened?"

"I guess I was eating too fast and a piece of chicken went down the wrong way."

"And—"

"I prayed to an angel and was able to get the food up. I always pray to him when I have serious challenges. And I send this angel to all my loved ones when they need help. I sent my angel to my granddaughter once when she needed a hand. I sent him to my son—to keep watch over his family."

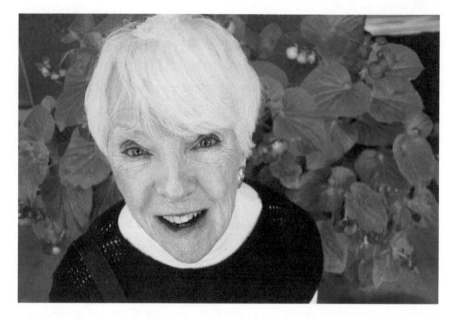

Arlene

I felt myself getting hopelessly behind in my afternoon clinic sched-ule, but Arlene's story was intriguing. I told myself to slow down, take a breath and listen.

"Arlene, this is fascinating. Tell me more. For starters, what angel do you call on in these situations?"

"My angel?"

"Yes."

"Why, he's your son. I call on Graham."

"My son?"

"Of course. I have been calling on him for the last five years."

"Arlene, I am stunned."

"Oh yes! Your son—he's been helping a lot of people."

Among Graham's inner circle of childhood pals was Alex Pecorella, a handsome, feisty kid with intense Mediterranean eyes. Alex was instinctively protective of his friend in the wheelchair and, despite the fact that Graham was nonverbal, the two became close during their early school years. After Graham went to Crotched, he and Alex saw less of one another, but, whenever they reconnected, the affection and trust born in early childhood remained strong. By the time Graham moved home at age twenty-two, Alex's family had moved to another state, and he was finishing college. He was an intense young man, but it surprised nearly everyone when he announced that he was joining the Marine Corps. Around the time of that momentous decision, he wrote about Graham in a letter to Cynthia:

> "I know that, in the coming years, while I try to navigate the terrain at Quantico and, who knows where else in the world, I will have a guide with me. Someone who can tell me where to go, what to do and how to not give up, no matter what... I know that I am going to need a right hand man."

Alex became a team leader in the 2nd Battalion 5th Marines and served with distinction overseas. I contacted him later, to ask him about his friendship with Graham. He replied with this note:

> "Graham always seemed to have a calming effect on me, which was rare when I was young. Our classmates respected me when I was with Graham, something I didn't feel when he wasn't there.
>
> Graham was different from everyone else, not because he had cerebral palsy, but because he made a choice, along with his parents, to not let CP affect the way he was going to live his

life. He was determined to play baseball, swim, hike, sail and travel. And to laugh, joke and successfully flirt with more girls than I ever thought possible.

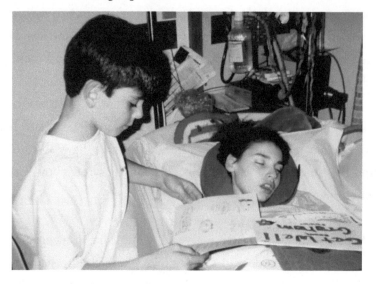

Alex with Graham at Children's Hospital.

Graham's life told a story of how to live regardless of the hand you are dealt, something it took me many more years to figure out. It is easy to fight when you know you are going to win, but to fight when your fate is unknown takes courage. It is easy to feel sorry for yourself when your combat load weighs eighty pounds, you are wet, sleep-deprived, and it's freezing cold. At that point, even a driven man starts to rationalize that he no longer can be the person he thought he could be. That is the point at which you start to draw on memories that help get you through.

For me, some of those memories are of Graham and how he would handle a difficult situation and face adversity. What would he think of me if he saw me give up?

Graham, I am eternally indebted to you for what you gave me. I will always tell your story. I will never leave you behind.

I will never give up because of you.

Your right hand man,

Alex"

When they were about ten years old, Graham's class went on a field trip. A speaker was addressing the group when Graham became restless and started to vocalize in a way that was disturbing the teacher and making the students uncomfortable. Ted Dimond, another of Graham's first friends, quietly put his arm around his companion and discreetly explained that it's not polite or wise to interrupt teachers. Graham quieted down. Even at the age of ten, Ted had intuitively assumed the role of advocate for his friend, probably before he even knew what the word meant. Ted Dimond, like Alex Pecorella and many of Graham's other classmates, grew up feeling comfortable around people who are different from them.

Years later, when I asked Ted about his friendship with Graham, he answered simply, "With Graham and me there was a nonverbal connection that I can't easily explain."

Ted Dimond went on to excel in athletics in secondary school and college, especially in lacrosse. He credits Graham with motivating him as an athlete. Apparently, seeing Graham working hard at simple tasks inspired Ted to work even harder to achieve his own "personal best" in competitive sports. In recognition of that influence, Ted wore the initials "GG" on his lacrosse helmet throughout his playing career. For a single-minded young athlete, that was the highest honor he could bestow on another person.

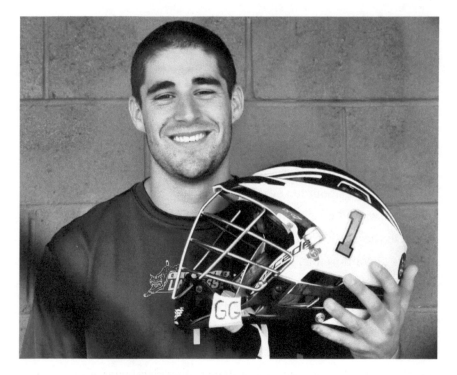

Ted

In the summer of 2011, Graham's fun-loving and steadfast counselors, Kaitlin, Maggie and Michelle, came up with the idea to create a garden in his memory at Camp Jabberwocky. Ultimately planted near the entrance to Camp, where it can be enjoyed by all who come and go, the garden contains native ferns, milkweeds and goldenrods and is edged by smooth beach stones. Before placing them around the garden, the stones were painted in playful designs by the campers and counselors. Through this living memorial, Graham's presence at Camp Jabberwocky is now eternal.

At the dedication of the garden, Kaitlin said,

"Graham was my secret keeper and still is, to this day. He was and is the person I turn to when I feel I have nowhere else to go. This garden is a testament to Graham's kind, quiet nature, his willingness to let others feel, and his acceptance of those feelings with no reservations. His garden is a way for all of us to heal and to become whole again.

Go to Graham's garden and leave happier than when you came. These rocks that we have been painting, and will continue to paint, represent the Jabberwocky love that encircles Graham and the love that Graham has for all of us."

Ross Lilly and our friends at AccesSportAmerica honored Graham's participation in its high-challenge water sports on Martha's Vineyard and on the Charles River in Boston by christening a boat in his name! Actually, the Hawaiian double-hulled canoe was named in honor of two young men. On the green port-side hull was the name *Graham*. On the yellow starboard-side hull was the name *Ángel*. Like Graham, Ángel had been an enthusiastic athlete in Ross's water sports programs despite a significant disability, and, like our son, Ángel had died young.

Graham was a boy of some privilege in the suburbs north of Boston, while Ángel was from an immigrant culture in the city. I suspected that Ross consciously chose to link Graham and Ángel in this unique way, as a reminder of our common humanity. Two hulls—when connected—create a single Hawaiian canoe. Although I never formally discussed this with Ross, Graham and Ángel's boat was clearly a metaphor. People who are different can create something strong and beautiful by working together. Their combined effort can move them both forward in a way that might not be possible for either one alone.

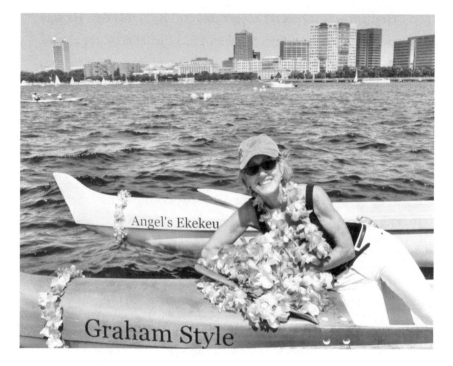

Cynthia with the canoe

On a calm early summer morning, against the backdrop of Boston's skyline, Ross gave a poignant remembrance of the two young men at a gathering on the Charles River. The Mayor's Cup Regatta is an annual series of rowing competitions that feature teams of paddlers, with and without disabilities, competing in a fleet of the big Hawaiian canoes. As the eager squads gathered on the banks of the Esplanade, the leafy urban park along the river that separates Boston and Cambridge, Ross introduced Cynthia and me to Ángel's family. For a few emotional moments, in fragments of Spanish and English, we shared our grief—and our pride.

As the sun began to melt away the early morning chill, Ross paid tribute to Graham and Ángel, finishing with these words:

"I like thinking of Graham and Ángel when I go to the dock and set up the equipment they used. The thought makes me put more energy and thought into the session, to honor them. It's the same with the other boats with names on them. Whenever I go out, I look at the names and try to think of the people with whom we travel. On this boat, Graham and Ángel are the aumakuas."

Ross hurried off to start the competition, leaving me to google that word on my cell phone. As *aumakuas,* in the ancient tradition of Hawaiian mysticism, Graham and Ángel are now the "ghosts of the ancestors" for all who paddle in their boat henceforth. Their spirits will energize and inspire those who follow them on the water, seeking friendship and an opportunity to challenge themselves.

When the races were finished, Ross, his family and the event's marvelous volunteers celebrated and laughed with the paddlers who were now sporting Hawaiian leis around their necks. The big gathering on the riverbank was diverse in every way. Some were elite athletes, including members of the Harvard University varsity football team, while others, in walkers and wheelchairs, had a range of serious disabilities. By design, each boat in the race had competed with crew members from both ends of that spectrum. As is the case wherever Ross and his colleagues gather people, the assorted participants in the Mayor's Cup Regatta that morning seemed to form a kind of community, one in which their differences had been diminished, blurred—or even erased.

As the festivities wound down, Ross addressed a group around Graham and Ángel's canoe. Departing from his familiar modus operandi of laughing and cracking jokes, he grew serious for a moment, articulating without apparent thought, the fundamental ethos of AccesSportAmerica: "The aumakuas of this boat, Graham and Ángel, will forever remind us that we are strong because we are on this journey together, and we do not leave anyone behind."

Jay Rothman, the Emmy-nominated producer of ESPN's *Monday Night Football*, heard about Graham's life from Cynthia, who was the stylist for the MNF broadcast team. When Jay learned that we were thinking of creating a Graham Hale Gardner Foundation, he came up with an idea for a kick-off event in Boston, volunteering to oversee the project on top of a grueling schedule that leaves him essentially without a day off for about half the year. Jay sensed that there was something highly unusual about the beautiful boy in the photos and stories that Cynthia shared with him. Although he never met Graham, Jay told us later that "Graham's spirit and strength helped me through a very rough time in my own life when my daughter was seriously ill, the most difficult time in my life."

Every member of the MNF broadcast team that year, including Mike Turico, Ron Jaworski, Jon Gruden, Michele Tafoya and Suzy Kolber jumped on board, working their connections to acquire coveted auction items, including autographed NFL helmets and jerseys. On a Saturday evening, before a Monday Night Football game between the Patriots and Jets, the MNF "talent" shared auctioneer duties. In front of a capacity gathering at The Greatest Bar on Friend Street in Boston's West End, they spiced their fundraising pitches with irreverent humor that would have been off-limits on the air. A nice sum of money was raised through the generosity of Graham's fans in attendance and his foundation was off to a roaring start. According to Jay, "It was an honor to rally for Graham, now and in the future."

After the rousing fundraiser, we were ready to officially launch the Graham Hale Gardner Foundation. It felt logical to kick off the organization's work by sponsoring one of the high-challenge sports that Graham loved. His Jabberwocky counselor and passionate friend, Michelle Moore, had been developing a plan to take a group of sixteen people from Camp with mixed abilities on a ski weekend in the White Mountains of New Hampshire. We asked Michelle if our new fund could help, and she excitedly agreed. The Graham Hale Gardner Foundation could not have asked for a more perfect beginning than to collaborate on a mixed-ability alpine adventure with a cherished Jabberwocky friend.

A date was set, and some acquaintances of Michelle's donated the use of an accessible farmhouse in Conway, New Hampshire. Cynthia cooked for the big group, once again featuring her signature challah French toast with maple syrup and fresh berries. I helped out at nearby Loon Mountain, where a team of high-spirited instructors from the Disabled Ski Program got our whole group, including campers in wheelchairs, to the top of the mountain.

We had an exhilarating day on high alpine trails lined by frosted fir trees. A gentle snowfall began and clouds limited visibility. But everyone in our group seemed to have a rousing athletic experience up there in the mist, with hoots of excitement periodically interrupting the muffled quiet of a big mountain in winter. It was marvelous to see friends ordinarily confined to wheelchairs descending challenging slopes, like Bear Claw and Flying Fox, riding sit skis with their instructors at speeds I struggled to keep up with. As remarkable as it was to see our Jabberwocky gang up there in the clouds at the top of Loon Mountain, Cynthia and I found ourselves amazed in a different way when the group returned to the rustic farmhouse after skiing. No special technologies or organized activities were needed to manufacture merriment for that bunch. Carefree mischief flowed from them quite naturally.

There was no television in the big living room. After the day's exertions, the sixteen old and new friends lay together on the floor and on beanbag chairs, laughing and teasing one another with no regard for political correctness. The ones who could physically do more assisted the ones who needed help in the completely natural manner of Camp Jabberwocky. Humorously indecent stories from the previous summer were shared with licentious flair during dinner. Later on, in lieu of bedtime stories, a counselor read whimsical verses from Lewis Carroll, the author of the quintessential nonsense poem "Jabberwocky," to which the camp owes its name. The collection of weary campers, counselors and friends chortled as she read:

"If I had a world of my own, everything would be nonsense. Nothing would be what it is, because everything would be what it isn't. And contrary wise, what is, it wouldn't be. And what it wouldn't be, it would. You see?"

Nearly everyone nodded.

Two summers after Graham passed away, Cynthia hailed a Yellow Cab in midtown Manhattan on a brilliant June morning. She engaged the driver in conversation in her natural friendly way. Through the streaked Plexiglas window separating them, she discerned weathered Slavic features. As her mind's eye, she pictured a strong peasant man in a field with horses and haystacks, the driver introduced himself in a thick Russian accent—Vladimir.

Through the little sliding window in the Plexiglas, Cynthia noticed what appeared to be a school photo of a boy about six years old in a display on the grimy dashboard and asked the cabbie who he was. With rising pride, Vladimir told her about his grandson, surprised that a well-heeled stranger would express an interest in his family.

When Cynthia came to her destination, she paid the driver and smiled at him. He looked intently at her and asked, "What about you, do you have children?"

Cynthia told him that her only child had passed away two and a half years earlier and that she and his father had been blessed to have such a boy for a son. She told Vladimir that she was not afraid to talk about Graham—it made her happy to talk about him. The Russian looked stunned. Like most people seeing a photograph of Graham for the first time, he found it hard to believe that Graham was profoundly disabled. After Cynthia told him a little about her son's life, the cabbie asked if there was a foundation or some other way that the boy was to be remembered. Cynthia briefly told him about our nascent foundation in Graham's honor and what it hoped to accomplish.

From his pocket, Vladimir produced a tattered leather wallet bulging with scraps of paper and business cards. He selected a wrinkled five-dollar bill, handed it to Cynthia with a kind look and wished her well. She asked for his name and address, which he scribbled on a torn scrap of paper. A few moments later, he pulled his cab into the teeming Manhattan traffic and was gone. Cynthia stood on the sidewalk for a moment, looking at the frayed bill and the Brooklyn address scribbled in unfamiliar Russian cursive. She was already mentally drafting the thank you note she would write to Vladimir when she got home.

Trying to get a handle on the concept of time usually ends up being an elusive exercise, unless you're a theoretical physicist. I bet some of them struggle with it, too. How long a time, for example, is twenty-two years, eleven months and three days? That was the question I pondered after visiting my friend Marie Montina, on the twenty-third floor of the Elison Building at MGH. Her room had spectacular views of the Charles River that was dotted with sailboats and collegiate crews from Harvard, MIT and Boston University in shiny rowing boats called shells. The city skyline to the west was silhouetted against a pale sunset of pink and orange.

Marie, a medical assistant at MGH who grew up in Haiti, wasn't thinking about the spectacular views of the river or the sunset. Her twin babies had been stillborn two days earlier. They would have been her first children—the triumphant culmination of years of yearning to have a family of her own. Her disbelief was acute and unfathomable. I knew there was nothing to say that wouldn't sound trite, but I was glad to be there with her for a little while and hold her hand with the solidarity of another parent who understood that kind of loss. As we sat for some time in silence, Marie's tragedy inevitably made me consider Cynthia's and mine. Graham's absence was fresh and exquisitely painful. Yet we had him with us for almost twenty-three years. Marie had held her children for just a couple of minutes, and then they were gone. Cynthia and I would continue to feel cheated by not having had Graham longer, but Marie's experience put ours in a different light.

I thought about a recent conversation I had with Dale Minor, the warmhearted New Hampshire social worker who had tried so hard to help us at the time of Graham's graduation from Crotched Mountain. When I told Dale that Graham had passed away, her response had been immediate: "It's not how long he was here, it's how much love he spread while he was here."

I stared out Marie's window at the river and the city below where life relentlessly carried on. The familiar red MBTA trains were carrying commuters and students across the Emerson Bridge to Cambridge. The clunky-looking amphibious duck boats were entertaining tourists on the river. Kids were playing baseball and soccer on the Esplanade, the verdant sliver of parkland that parallels the river along Boston's Back Bay. Life was simply going on, oblivious to the indescribable loss that Marie was experiencing. I watched the river where it widens near the Museum of Science and realized that I had once sat in a power boat on that exact spot and watched Graham windsurfing with AccesSportAmerica.

Marie and I shared tears and a long hug before I left. I knew that my friend would be discharged the next day into a world that would seem indifferent to her terrible loss.

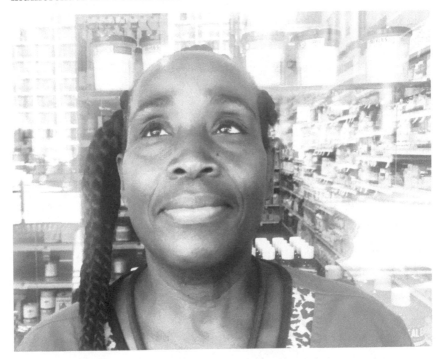

Marie

I stepped into the big Elison elevator and found myself watching the diverse faces avoiding eye contact in the confined space. As patients, families and caregivers got on and off during the stop-and-go ride to the lobby, it occurred to me that the entire spectrum of human emotion could be riding in that single car. Someone may have been experiencing the stunning euphoria of learning that they were cancer-free. Someone else might have just received the worst news of their life. The smiling senior couple may have come to welcome a new family member into the world. And one of those people might have just said goodbye to the person they loved more than anyone else in the world.

On his birthday, two years after he passed away, the kindhearted Marble-head neighbors and friends who had embraced him and celebrated him since his childhood, dedicated a living memorial to Graham. At the edge of a twelve-acre nature preserve called the Goldthwait Reservation, next to a path to the beach that Cynthia and Graham had traveled together hundreds of times, they planted a beautiful and unusual tree to honor Graham. The tree is a witch hazel whose bright yellow flowers resemble shredded sunbursts. Its unusual feature is that it can start blooming late in the harsh New England winter and keep its blossoms until early March, the time of Graham's birthday. The tree was planted in a sacred place for Cynthia and Graham, the special spot where their walks began and ended, next to the sweeping salt marsh protected from the Atlantic by a massive wall of rounded beach stones.

Jean Verbridge, Susie Ryan and Margaret Bacon were among the special friends who conceived of this tribute and took great pains to place it in harmony with its unique setting. Those neighbors had been vehement advocates for Graham throughout his life and, at the dedication, shared their reflections about him, as did a number of other friends who were with us that day. A few weeks later, Susie and Russell Ryan implausibly collected a beach rock the size of a rugby ball and had Graham's name engraved on it. They placed it at the base of the witch hazel tree, where those who knew Graham can think about him as they make their way to and from the beach. It also occurred to Susie and Russell that visitors who never met Graham and were new to that enchanted place might see the stone and wonder, "Who was he?"

About a month later, Cynthia was in the Goldthwait area to participate in a neighborhood cleanup on a Sunday morning. A neighbor mentioned that her four-year-old daughter, Meredith, was fascinated by the tree and rock. Cynthia picked up the youngster and brought her over to the memorial to tell her about Graham. Cynthia had kissed the rock with red lipstick when Susie and Russell first placed it there, and the voluptuous lip marks were still visible. Meredith asked Cynthia if she had put her lips on the rock. Cynthia replied that she did, just as she had kissed Graham—hundreds of times a day. Cynthia wrote this to me about the memorial:

"It's the most beautiful place. I'm often there at 5:30 a.m. when the moon and stars are still in the sky and the sun is on the horizon. The wind is blowing and you can hear the ocean. It was a perfect place for Graham because he loved the elements with such a passion. Now he's embracing all who come to this little corner of the world that we frequented.

I used to take him to the top of the boardwalk before we left for Crotched Mountain on Mondays and when we returned. I'd tell him how lucky we were and to look around and drink it all in.

This was his backyard which he should etch in his memory and draw from all week. I'd say, 'God willing, Bud, we'll be back here soon.' I always told him how fortunate we were to have each other, you, our home and our friends and family.
Every time he left my arms, I would remind him."

Shortly after the dedication of the memorial to Graham, Cynthia and I found an additional surprise at the base of the witch hazel tree. Surrounding the big stone with Graham's name on it, smaller heart-shaped beach rocks had appeared. They had been placed in the soft earth there with care by unknown individuals. There were just a few at first, but within several weeks, there were dozens of them—stone hearts of different sizes, colors and textures. New heart-shaped stones appear at the base of Graham's witch hazel tree from time to time, even now.

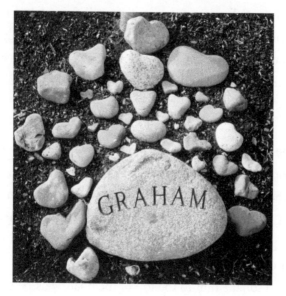

Cynthia was walking among the rounded beach stones at Goldthwait and stopped at a weathered picnic table. It was the special place where she had so often fed Graham his dinner, overlooking the Atlantic in all of its wildly different moods.

She was surprised to see an Indian couple walking together slowly into the choppy water where we had scattered some of Graham's ashes a year earlier. It seemed curious that they were wading into the surf fully clothed in traditional East Indian garments. Then she understood. The couple was carrying a small bag. As the delicate young woman became progressively soaked by wind-swept waves, her partner emptied the container into the surf. The woman, intuitively recognized by Cynthia as a mother, remained motionless with her hand over her heart. The quantity of ashes was small, consistent with the remains of a child. Cynthia watched the scene play out directly in front of her, in the very place that she and Graham had shared so passionately.

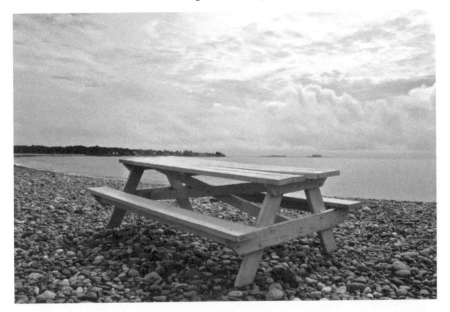

She spoke to Graham and asked him to welcome this person whose earthly remains were now intertwined with his in the waters off Marblehead. As she moved away from the beach with the poignant scene imprinted in her heart, she spoke to Graham once again and asked him, as we have done many times now, for a sign—that the soul who had been taken from his parents would be OK. That the mother and the father would be OK. That he, Graham, was okay and that Cynthia and I would be OK. As her gaze absently moved across the horizon, she noticed a lone cloud in the cornflower blue sky.

It was shaped like a heart.

EPILOGUE

On a sabbatical from my career at MGH, I helped out at the Adaptive Ski School in Vail, Colorado, for a winter. Working among adults and kids with disabilities and their helpers was familiar and uplifting. Joyful memories of tethering Graham in his sit ski frequently flooded my emotions. One night I wrote my son a note, hoping it would reach him across the mysteries of time and space:

"Dear Bud,

I wish you could see all this. The sun-splashed groves of aspen trees. Majestic ponderosa pines reaching for the cobalt blue sky that merges with infinity beyond the sawtooth peaks of the Continental Divide.

I wish you could hear the whirring of the shivs as the chairlift passes over its massive stanchions, the crunching of spring snow under ski boots, the swishing sound of skis carving arcs in the snow and the hoots of dear friends as they dance with this majestic mountain.

I wish you could smell the pleasing scent of paraffin wax being ironed onto the bases of our skis, the succulent aroma of chicken and burgers in the rarified air outside Two Elk Lodge and the pungent fragrance of piñon pine being burned at night in wood fires in lodges in the village.

I wish you could feel the warmth of the sun on your face this much closer to heaven and the pleasant glow of sore muscles after a day on the big mountain.

And I wish you could feel my arms hugging you in this special place. I am so sorry that you could not experience all of this with me.

Or did you?"

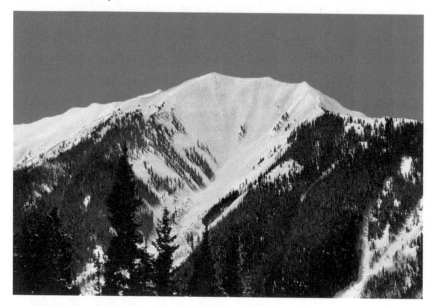

AFTERWORD

"If the sun were to explode you wouldn't even know about it for eight minutes because that's how long it takes for light to travel from the sun to the earth."
—Jonathan Safran Foer,
Extremely Loud and Incredibly Close

When I finished writing these stories, the exhilaration that I expected was tempered by an empty feeling. Perhaps the writing was my eight minutes in the sun, and I didn't want them to end. In the stories, I emphasized the light that Graham shone on our world and, perhaps subconsciously, chose not to dwell on our darker experiences, like his epilepsy. During his seizures, Graham's body jerked violently, the color drained from his face, and he stopped breathing for agonizing seconds. He bit his tongue and lips. Despite medication, those convulsions happened hundreds of times and each one was harrowing.

Even during sustained periods without seizures, Graham often appeared physically uncomfortable. As his de facto physician for most of his life, I was never able to find an explanation for that discomfort, leaving me chronically worried that I might be missing a serious medical problem. Or, was I missing the possibility that Graham was in physical pain? Over the years, sleep deprivation was a frequent stressor for all of us. Graham's sleep patterns were interrupted by involuntary movements, muscle spasticity and whatever it was that made him so uncomfortable at times. The lack of refreshing sleep was traumatic. We lived with disrupted sleep for years, at times intensifying friction between Cynthia and me.

When Graham was away from home, we feared what a predator might do to a beautiful boy who could not speak. At his residential school, we knew his regular helpers very well, and they were never far from him. But, occasionally, one would call in sick and a male aide we had never met would fill in for her. That person would undress Graham and bathe him in a closed shower room. We had to trust that the school had vetted those individuals carefully.

Dealing with Graham's disability was undeniably difficult. People wondered how we did it—constantly lifting him, feeding him, bathing him and changing his "briefs." It *was* difficult, and many people assumed that it must be a burden that was hard to bear. But, honestly, caring for Graham never felt like a burden to Cynthia and me. Loving someone that much seemed to give us strength. And when we did feel depleted, we looked to Graham for guidance and, in his unique way, he helped us find reserves of physical and spiritual energy.

Cynthia and I joked with our friends who had "normal" children that *we* actually had it easy. We never had to worry about Graham cracking up the car! We never had to bail him out of jail for being drunk and disorderly! Shoplifting was highly unlikely! And he never railed about what pathetic parents we were.

When I speak to groups of medical students and even seasoned doctors, I often refer to this familiar Shakespearean passage from *The Merchant of Venice* when discussing the special gift of being a caregiver:

"The quality of mercy is not strained.
It droppeth as the gentle rain from heaven
Upon the place beneath. It is twice blest:
It blesses him that gives and him that takes."

Cynthia and I felt blessed to care for Graham. And through him, we met people who were inspired by the "quality of mercy" in ways we could never have imagined were possible. At Zeno Mountain Farm there are wheelchair-accessible treehouses! The campers and counselors of Camp Jabberwocky create original musicals each summer! Graham opened the door to this astonishing world, and in it we discovered heroes who changed how we thought about life itself. One was Dr. Harry Webster, the Tufts University pediatric rehabilitation specialist, who would phone us out of the blue on major holidays.

"Hello Cynthia and Steven. I'm sitting in my office looking through some charts and a snapshot of Graham just fell out. How is the young superstar doing these days?"

"Harry, thank you so much for checking in! He's doing great. Are you aware that it's Christmas Eve?"

As the years passed, Cynthia and I were continually astonished by people like Harry, "the ones who give," including therapists, teachers, aides, friends, neighbors and, of course, the camp counselors. All of those people passionately assisted Graham during his lifetime.

At the same time, we were stunned by the "ones who receive," the resilient people we met with disabilities who were the recipients of all that "gentle rain." People like Shirley Lewis and Patty Keleher, Jabberwocky campers who have severe forms of cerebral palsy—and simply cannot stop smiling.

"Time will ease your pain," people say. But sometimes I think I actually preferred living with the acute pain of losing Graham—when my emotions were raw and there was nothing but love in my consciousness. I understand that all things fade in time, but I wish that were not true with regard to the life we had with Graham. Even some of our most exquisite memories are somewhat muted now. I walk through Graham's room occasionally without even thinking of him. For me, there will never be another journey that will compare to the experience of being Graham's father. I sometimes wonder why I am still here, when no awakening, no anguish, no joy, no love will compare with what I experienced with him.

Wherever he is, Cynthia and I love Graham right now just as much as ever. If our feelings for him are the same, then he must still love us just as much across the unknowable dimensions that presently separate us. A comforting notion. One thing we know with certainty is that Graham would want us to embrace the message on the memorial card handed out at the celebration of his life:

"Now go out and love some more."

In that spirit, I return each summer as a doctor at Camp Jabberwocky. Cynthia volunteers throughout the year at the equally magical Zeno Mountain Farm. We love to be among people who are resilient and fun— Graham's kind of people. In the end, Cynthia and I simply miss our son. We miss everything about him, but especially hugging him, stroking his silky hair and telling him—for the millionth time—how much we love him.

Sometimes, in bed at night, I am able to quiet my mind and allow it to drift back to the time when Graham came home. I think of that as my six weeks of heaven on earth. I wonder if I will ever experience that feeling again. Graham and I often listened to Kenny Loggins' tender version of

"Somewhere Out There" on the album *House at Pooh Corner.* The sentimental song was written for *An American Tail,* the animated musical adventure film about a family of Russian mice that emigrates by boat from Imperial Russia to the United States in search of freedom. Fievel, the family's young son, falls overboard in a violent storm and is lost at sea. Miraculously, Fievel survives. But he finds himself alone in America with no way to find his family. The song captures the yearning for one another that he and his parents feel—not knowing if they will ever see one another again.

> *"Somewhere out there*
> *Beneath the pale moonlight*
> *Someone's thinking of me*
> *And loving me tonight*
> *Somewhere out there*
> *Someone's saying a prayer*
> *That we'll find one another*
> *In that great somewhere out there*
> *Somewhere out there*
> *If love can see us through*
> *Then we'll be together*
> *Somewhere out there*
> *Out where dreams come true."*

Happily, at the conclusion of *An American Tail,* Fievel is reunited with his family. A Hollywood ending. Friends of mine believe that Graham will be the first one to greet me when my own time comes to "cross over."

Will you, my beloved boy?

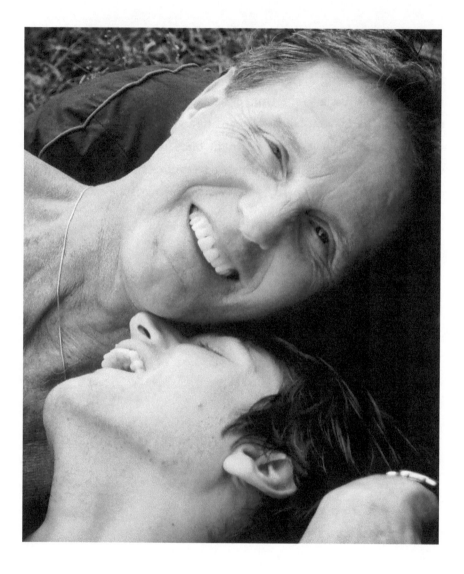

APPENDIX ONE:

THE GRAHAM HALE GARDNER ANGEL AWARD

On a blustery day in September of 2010, the inaugural Graham Hale Gardner Angel Award was presented to Cynthia and me on our son's behalf by Spaulding Rehabilitation Hospital. The ceremony was held at the hospital's sun-splashed pier on the Charles River in Boston as part of a community celebration that featured live music, food tastings from local restaurants, a silent auction and carnival activities for kids. The spirited gathering watched as patients from the hospital—some normally in wheelchairs—launched special windsurfers from the dock and paddled out on the calm waters of the river. Each of those courageous people was carefully assisted by an instructor from AccesSportAmerica, kneeling or standing on the board with them. Against the backdrop of the city skyline, we marveled as adults and children with significant medical conditions raised sails and caught the wind where the river widens into a tranquil basin between Boston and Cambridge.

It was in that sparkling place a few years earlier, emboldened by his mom, that Graham had been one of the first youngsters with a significant disability to serve as a kind of test pilot for the windsurfing program.

At the time, the notion that participation in high-challenge sports could enhance recovery from illness or injury was—figuratively and literally—an idea in the wind.

The award that was established in Graham's honor was the brainchild of the hospital's leaders, particularly the irrepressible Steven Patrick, along with an exuberant Spaulding advocate named Jane Weingarten. Inspired by the legacy of her late husband, Dr. Charles Weingarten, Jane was an early believer in the therapeutic potential of adaptive sports. Since that breezy day on the Spaulding waterfront in 2010, the award that "honors Graham's adventurous spirit and exuberant love of life" has been presented annually to a disabled athlete, instructor or caregiver. The award winners are a stunning group of people who personify resilience while caring deeply about improving the lives of others.

Besides windsurfing, a growing number of athletic activities sponsored by Spaulding are now available to both hospital patients and people with disabilities throughout New England. Many challenge themselves with sports that can be intimidating even for the able-bodied, including snow skiing. Liberated from the confines of hospital wards and clinics—outdoors in the light of day—some of these spirited people rediscover a precious sense of freedom that might have seemed forever lost. For much of the year, it is not unusual to spot the Spaulding athletes paddling canoes on Boston Harbor and waving to tugboat captains, or riding adapted bikes on paths along the waterfront—often moving considerably faster than the nearby automobiles! For people who summon the nerve to participate in adaptive sports, the rewards are often profound, including enhanced self-esteem and renewed optimism about what is possible for them in the future.

Outside, in the wind and ever-changing New England weather, an additional prize awaits those athletes: the healing elixir of laughing with other people who are figuratively—and sometimes literally—in the same boat.

Here are a few words about the inspirational recipients of the Graham Hale Gardner Angel Award.

2011. The Lilley Family

I hope you recall my descriptions of Ross Lilley, the playful, charismatic protagonist in the stories called *Sengekontacket, Chilmark* and *Aumakuas*. Ross was the first person to develop adaptive windsurfing in the United States. Assisted by his wife Jean, daughter Hanna, and son Josh, he created the innovative program called AccesSportAmerica that would ultimately open the door to a wide variety of high-challenge sports—on and off the water—for people with disabilities of all ages. In addition to his pioneering work in adaptive sports at Spaulding and elsewhere, Ross is an ordained minister with another mission that I have witnessed with fascination over many years—to break down the differences that separate people and bring them closer together in a community of mutual support, laughter and hope.

2012. David Leone

This Dartmouth-educated geologist is an environmentalist and consultant in hazardous waste cleanup. After suffering a spinal cord injury in a fall from a ladder at his home, Dave underwent surgery at a Boston hospital before being transferred to Spaulding for rehabilitation. His wife Michele was pregnant, and the couple became parents for the first time during Dave's arduous months there. During that time he became one of the first patients with a spinal cord injury to use a training tool called a "Functional Electrical Stimulation Rowing Device." Dave's competitive spirit was demonstrated when he set—and still holds—the world adaptive record for 1,000 meters on that indoor rowing apparatus. He continues to be involved in Spaulding's ExPD program (Exercise for Persons with Disabilities), which designs challenging exercise programs for appropriate patients with spinal cord injuries and neurological conditions like ALS. After his hospitalization, Dave made a seminal decision—"to go home and live my life." Today, among other passions, he rides the roads of Massachusetts using a hand cycle and coaches his son's soccer team.

2013. Jamie Bemis

Jamie Bemis worked as a teacher and professional baker before starting "Gaining Ground," a nonprofit enterprise whose volunteers grow fresh produce for homeless shelters in the Boston area. She and her husband John created vegetable gardens that are elevated several feet above ground level, making them accessible to workers in wheelchairs. In 2011, Jamie suffered a serious stroke, paralyzing her right side. At Spaulding, she experienced what she calls "tough love," painstakingly learning to walk again before riding a bike and, ultimately, driving a car. Jamie credits adaptive sports for playing a significant role in reclaiming a joyful and dynamic life.

She devotes much of her time now to philanthropy and made a generous donation to Spaulding for the purpose of studying, in a scientific way, the therapeutic benefit of adaptive sports. About thirty athletic activities are being investigated now, including rock wall climbing, wheelchair dance and seated volleyball. Inspired, in part, by Jamie, Spaulding and its affiliates also sponsor "Sport and Spirit" weekends for wounded military veterans.

2014. The Levine Family

It's challenging enough for a mother and father to contend with one child with a significant neurologic disorder, but the Levine family is managing with two. Shaina, now fifteen, was diagnosed with cerebral palsy at thirteen months of age, after birth complications. Samuel, now fourteen, had a seizure three days after his birth. He, too, was diagnosed with CP. Their parents, Laurence and Samantha, embarked on a stunning odyssey, leaving their home in South Africa with the singular goal of finding the best possible care for their children, no matter where it might take them in the world. Shaina and Samuel were seen by specialists in numerous cities in Europe and the U.S., as emotionally and physically taxing months turned into years. Shaina struggled with breathing troubles caused by issues with her respiratory muscles and tightness in her leg muscles required a series of painful surgeries. Samuel's neurologic difficulties were somewhat different, but he continually grappled with weakness and tightness in the muscles on one side of his body.

In the summer of 2013, the Levine family arrived in Boston where Samuel underwent a nine-hour orthopedic surgery at Boston Children's Hospital. Postoperatively, he was transferred to Spaulding Hospital's futuristic new home on Boston Harbor. From the enormous windows of his room on the eighth floor, he could see patients who were recovering from surgeries and injuries—outside in the sunshine, working with their therapists. To Samuel's surprise, some of the patients were out on the water in colorful canoes and kayaks.

Shaina, meanwhile, had come to Boston to begin a new phase of her own therapy, working with a "hand-cycle" under the guidance of Spaulding's athletic trainers. In his initial postoperative days—still confined to a hospital bed—Samuel saw his sister's face beaming with pride after her sessions with the adaptive sports team. Just two months after his surgery, on a chilly fall afternoon, Samuel stood with assistance and helped sail a windsurfer across Boston Harbor.

Those of us who are caregivers know that we enjoy a privileged—even sacred—relationship with patients and families. On occasion, each of us has interacted with people so inspiring that we are left to wonder who is getting more out of the relationship—is it the patient or is it me? That question has occurred to nearly every doctor, nurse, therapist, athletic trainer and administrator who has interacted with the Levine family.

Spaulding's motto is "Find Your Strength." Samuel, Shaina and their parents have found strength, with the passionate assistance of the caregivers and administrators of Spaulding Hospital. It may be equally true, however, that the Levine family has helped the people privileged to assist them to discover new strengths of their own. In Samantha's words, both Samuel and Shaina are now "well on their way to a brighter and more abled future."

2015. Cheri Blauwet, MD

After a childhood spinal cord injury in Iowa confined her to a wheelchair, Cheri Blauwet showed her strength of character by becoming an elite athlete, earning a gold medal at the Paralympics in Athens and winning the New York City Marathon, Wheelchair Division (twice), the Boston Marathon (twice) and the Los Angeles Marathon (four times).

After attending the Stanford University School of Medicine, she completed residency and fellowship training in Boston and joined the faculty at Harvard Medical School. She specializes in sports medicine, while serving in many leadership and advocacy roles for people with disabilities, nationally and internationally. This petite force of nature, much-loved among her patients and colleagues at Spaulding and the medical school, embodies the spirit of a caregiver. In 2015, she was chosen to speak on the floor of the United Nations on the International Day of Sport for

Development and Peace. Among numerous other leadership positions, she currently serves on the Board of Directors of the International Olympic Committee.

And she recently became a mother.

2016. The Miller Family

The Miller family has a multigenerational connection with Spaulding and its adaptive sports programs. The relationship began many years ago when Oscar Miller received post-op treatment at Spaulding and was amazed by the care he received. He and his wife Lee decided to provide support as the hospital explored the idea of adaptive sports as a component of rehabilitation. A connection grew between the family and the forward-thinking hospital executives who sensed the potential of athletic activities in helping patients to regain function after trauma. When Oscar passed away, Lee passionately carried on the family's support.

Later, the Miller's son, Gary, joined Spaulding's Development Committee and continues to zealously support the hospital's mission of restoring people to their highest function possible, to "find their strength." Gary's wife, Arlene, describes Spaulding as "a big, extended family that begins with the greeters at the front desk." For generations, she says, the Miller family has been amazed by "the incredible number of people who are helped by this remarkable place."

2017. Meredith Koch

On the day before her birthday in 2015, a recreational skier and volunteer EMT named Meredith Koch was assisting some friends, who were moving an upright piano off the bed of a pickup truck near Burlington, Vermont. The piano lurched unexpectedly and landed on the young woman, fracturing her sternum and crushing part of her lumbar spine. After nine hours of surgery, she woke up in an ICU paralyzed from the waist down. On the operating table, she turned twenty-five years old. A source of inspiration for Meredith during her lengthy rehabilitation was a remarkable woman she had only read about, Dr. Cheri Blauwet. Eventually, the women would meet and become friends.

Less than a year after the accident, Meredith began to ski again. After falling repeatedly while seated on a mono ski at Loon Mountain in New Hampshire, she famously stated, "I will not let a piano stop me from doing something I love!" That resilience and her message of hope and inclusion have since inspired professional and lay audiences through presentations including the TED talk she gave in Newport, Rhode Island. Meredith still uses crutches, but she can walk short distances now without them, using only light braces on her lower legs. She works at a biomedical engineering company that develops innovative technologies for the health sciences. Besides skiing, she has tackled adaptive rock climbing and surfing.

Aquatic therapy, however, has become a key component of Meredith's rehabilitation and, after countless hours in the pool, swimming is her new passion. Nobody who has met Meredith finds it surprising that, in her words, "My new dream is to swim in the Paralympics for Team USA."

2018. Edna Sears

Throughout her life, an indomitable woman named Edna Sears has had a love affair with ice hockey. Now ninety-four years old, she has been a prominent force behind the growth of adaptive hockey programs in Eastern Massachusetts. For decades, Edna and her late husband attended every hockey game played by Harvard's varsity teams. The couple found something magical in the *kish kish* sound of skate blades, the sharp *smack* of pucks hitting sticks and the fluid harmony of athletes gliding in arcs on an icy stage. But, over time, Edna became troubled that the boards around hockey rinks were figurative and literal barriers to people with disabilities. She decided to do something about it, setting a goal of allowing "people of all abilities to discover this wonderful sport."

Working with the Spaulding Adaptive Sports Program and other groups, including the US National Amputee Hockey Team, Edna became a sponsor of sled hockey programs in the Boston area. It was important to her that adults and children were welcome to join the teams, whether they had stopped playing hockey due to injury or were completely new to the sport. Thanks to Edna, the grinding *whoosh* of sled runners cutting through ice and the *thwack* of pucks connecting with hockey sticks are growing increasingly common at rinks throughout Eastern Massachusetts.

Brian Bardell, whose leg was amputated after being diagnosed with a liposarcoma, told the Boston Globe: "I have played sports all my life, and the thought of not being to play again was crushing. Thanks to sled hockey, it's an incredible feeling to be part of a team again, to get off the ice dripping with sweat, and not be able to wait to come back."

2019. Kristen McCosh

After a diving accident resulted in a spinal cord injury at age fifteen, Kristen has used a wheelchair. But that physical disability never dimmed her optimism or determination to lead a full and joyful life. After graduating from college, Kristen developed a growing calling as an advocate for individuals with disabilities and now leads Boston's Commission for Persons with Disabilities. In that capacity, Kristen's strong voice for inclusion and accessibility has dramatically impacted the actions of government and business leaders. The high hopes written into the 1990 Americans with Disabilities Act (ADA) are ever closer to becoming societal norms now, thanks to the message of empowerment embodied by Kristen. Disabled residents of Boston, and across the country, lead more independent lives and experience more fully all that their communities have to offer today, thanks to the ability of this remarkable woman to challenge assumptions and open doors.

APPENDIX TWO

CONDOLENCES

A mong the scores of condolences we received after Graham's death were these:

Your life has a kind of nobility because of Graham. You did all you could and worked hard to be the right father for him in every possible way. — Helen M.

Cynthia, you were a trailblazer and a model for us all. — Libby M.

You and Cynthia gave him all the opportunities for a wonderful and meaningful life. — Paul R.

No boy was ever more beloved by his father. In a world that aches for fathers who love their sons, I have never seen the like. The great love of your life, he is irreplaceable. — Gina H.

Cynthia, it was an incredible experience to see you with him. You could see his joy. — Kit

He brought out the best in you and everyone he touched. — Kate O.

Cynthia, you motivated me to be a better parent every time I saw you with Graham. — Jamie K.

He was a lucky, lucky child to have you as a father. — Bev B.

Graham's heart was surely bursting with love. — Cynthia R.

It was no wonder where Graham got his great perseverance with a mother like Cynthia. — James R.

He was such a wonderfully gentle soul. I so enjoyed watching his connection with you, an incredible father. — Kim H.

Words cannot express our sadness. He brought us so much love. Just his presence changed the mood of a room. We will forever carry our "inner Graham" within us. May God bless him. He is free. You both made an amazing human being. The strength and endurance he showed has humbled us forever. — Jenna S.

Your angel is now up in heaven watching over you. — Felicity G.

Your love and devotion show in your photographs. — Henry and Flo

I cry for you. — Leslie H.

Live this year with love, as Graham taught us all. — Barbara P.

He was a gift of pure, absolute, innocent love. — Marsha S.

You did so much for him and he gave back to you in equal measure. — Alex P. and Anita G.

God will embrace and love him until the time you are together again. — Pat M.

Graham is being welcomed in his new home with the open loving arms of your loved ones already there before him. — Ann Marie S.

He was a living angel. — Joanne G.

The wonderful picture of you and Graham hugging and smiling is indelibly imprinted in my head and heart. — Ellen

Jabberwocky will never be the same without him. — Suzanne R.

He was a remarkable, inspirational, extraordinary man who profoundly touched all who crossed his path. I could see and feel his courage and love. I could feel his joy. — Ellen S.

The way you cared for Graham, the way you showed your love, the

enjoyment he gave you—any of these would have been extraordinary—but you did it all—amazing! — Bayla C.

He was a beautiful and courageous boy. — Lisa H.

I am so sorry for the loss of your precious son. — Nancy B.

It was always so clear how much you loved him. — Jackie W.

Thank you for helping to create the most beautiful person that I've ever had the honor to know. He changed my life forever. — Kate F.

Graham left his mark on this world of ours. — Oswald M.

I cannot find the words. — Laurie O.

We will always remember your devotion and pride in your wonderful son. Graham opened up my eyes and taught me how to be more loving and caring. — Tina Q.

Please be comforted to know that love is eternal. — Sookie C.

He was such a great reminder of what can happen when so much love is given and absorbed and how important kindness is. — Lucille G.

You have moved us all so much, with your love of Graham, of family and of Camp Jabberwocky. — Nancy and Russ B.

I know how much your son impacted your life. It has been through you that so many people, such as me, have benefited from your compassion and care. For that, I thank your son. — Richard B.

It was your indomitable celebration of Graham, even when conditions made it very difficult, that I and many others at Camp realized should be the ruling philosophy for our camper/counselor relationships. — Gillian B.

I hope and pray that God takes the pieces of your hearts and mends them with your treasured memories. — Marylou B.

Thank you for sharing Graham with the world. — Kelsey G.

I have been praying for you every day and night since hearing of your loss. — Valerie

Although I never met your son, it is so evident that he was a vessel full

of Divine Life ... so eager to communicate it, without a word, to so many. — Jennifer P.

I was deeply inspired by the incredibly strong bond between you and Graham. — Cora S.

He will always be in your heart and inspire you to live on with hope, strength and grace, as he did. — Eileen P.

The magic and joyous memories of Graham are forever. — Priscilla *We are so deeply sorry to have lost such a great young man with a huge heart.* — Dawn M.

Graham was blessed to have a father like you and you were equally blessed to have such a wonderful son. — Jason L.

The warmth of your love for Graham warmed your entire home. Your devotion and delight in your son were so evident. — Melissa B.

Few have been granted the capacity to love so deeply.—Dawn *Graham's life was extremely impressive, but so too was his parents' devotion to him.* — Norman B.

He was so well loved and cared for. His eyes showed how much he understood. — Jean R.

It's not the years we spend on earth, but the love we share while we're here. — Dale M.

You two shared so many of life's wonders with Graham and showered him with love and adventure. — Marsha F.

I hope your heart is open to let your family, friends and patients care for you now. — Tom G.

What a beautiful life the two of you had together. You were the most wonderful, loving father. — Beth P.

This world is a better place because of people like him and also his parents. I will now go out and love some more. — John V.

There was this moment at the service, after people began sharing memories, when we felt the room fill up with a presence that can only be described as love. — Sidney M. and Margaret K.

I was blessed to be in his life, to know him and love him. — Fatou N.

Now you have an angel watching over you. — Roxanne G.

He was a bright light in a needy world. — Eleanor E.

Not many things in this world are perfect, but God's placement of Graham in your care was as close as anything gets. An amazing father, an amazing boy. — Lucille G.

I know how much you loved your son. — Jay H.

Graham brought an incomparable light and love to so many people. — Gwen R.

Knowing Graham was one of my life's highest honors. — Lisa

Our hearts are with you, aching over the loss of this marvelous human being. — MGH Beacon Hill Primary Care Staff

You and he were a joy to watch … the love and devotion you gave each other were inspiring and poignant. He was a gift from God. — Caroline E.

How proud you should both be for the fine man he became. — Priscilla H.

You are such a kind and gentle soul—I imagine Graham possessed many of those qualities that make you such a special man and trusted doctor. — Erin

When he died, he was with the person he loved the most, doing what he loved to do. — Roslyn B.

I know how devoted you were to him and the profound effect he had on your work and art. — Gene B.

Graham enjoyed the competition of who hugged and kissed him more. — Lisa P.

I only saw LOVE in your home. — Fatou N.

We feel that we have been emotionally attached to him for many years through your wonderful stories of him and his life. — Anne R.

Graham, a handsome, proud young man packed everything into his life with the support of his fine parents. — Sara

If only every child born was loved and enjoyed the way Graham was— what a world this would be. — Norma

Graham, you will never know how you changed me. — Merrill P.

Your love for him was so great and true. — Jean K.

I will choose to believe that when he left this life, Graham walked strong and confident into another one filled with Light, once again shining on him. — Marilyn F.

You cherished your son and he nourished you. — Barbara P.

Your love, patience and faith in Graham provided him with a joyful and dignified life. — Linda W.

His short life was so full because of how you shared yours with him. — Suzi N.

He left the world doing what he loved the most with his dad. — Barb

Graham is forever frozen in our lives as a beautiful, loving young man. — Barbara P.

We all grew, simply by knowing him. — Blake A.

It was an honor to be at the service. I never met Graham, but I can now say that Graham has affected my life. — Lock W.

What has come through above all else has been your true and genuine love for him. — John B.

I did not know your son. But I know of your life and your love of this precious human being. His life, his story and his loss are extraordinary. — Regina

What an inspiring young man. A perfectly beautiful person, both inside and out. — Sandra

His ability to remain selfless, despite challenges most of us will never face, truly inspired me. — James R.

You and he gave a profound living gift to the rest of us: I guarantee there

is more kindness, gentleness, appreciation, gratitude and hope in the world today because of Graham's life. — Chip R.

A heart can speak louder than words and eyes can shine with love. — Lynn G.

The entire universe is a brighter place because of you, Graham. — Betsy P.

If you wanted to know what an angel looks like or to see heaven, all you had to do was look into Graham's eyes. I became one of his caregivers, but the real giver was Graham. — Nancy G.

Graham's spirit has always been an inspiration to us. We admire his courage. We are so grateful to know him, to hold onto his big smile and to remember our friend. — H.G.

His happiness was a tribute to you as parents. The Lord has Graham under his special watch and love. — Pat M.

I did not know Graham, but his obituary was the most beautiful tribute I've ever seen. — Marjorie

I did not know your son. But I know of your life and your love for this precious human being. His life, his story, his loss are extraordinary. My deepest sympathies to all who loved him. — An RN

Graham was the one who taught me how powerfully healing a touch could be. He gave me a sense of serenity when I was with him. — Renee

Over a decade has passed since I spent time as Graham's helper at his Marblehead summer camp, but I still remember his smile, his patience and his light. — Charlotte M.

He came from you and his life, its beauty and influence, lives within you. — Cynthia

Cynthia is amazing. She is so strong. I saw them jogging every day. How did she do it? — Suzy N.

Graham's childhood buddies have him in their lives every day. He is part of their sensitivity to all things different and wonderful. — Russell R.

Cynthia, every child would crave the kind of love you represent. Every child should know the feeling of being kissed awake in the morning. — Katie R.

You raised a tender and caring boy who truly enriched other people's lives and thus the world. — Gwen R.

That light, that love is not diminished. — Susan R.

Graham knew the sounds and smell of the wind and the sea as he glided along the streets of Marblehead. He knew acceptance and friendship. He knew the loving voice of his mother talking to him as an equal. In summary, Cynthia, Graham only knew love. The ultimate gift. — Jeannette

He informs every beat of your heart. — Gina

Thank you for exemplifying the power of a mother's love. — Carrie S.

Cynthia, there was nothing but love in your house and, clearly, you and Graham surrounded one another with it every moment you spent together. — Marise H.

When I look at his photos, I can tell that he has an amazing sense of the love that was around him. — Martha

I was profoundly moved by the depth of your love and unwavering commitment to Graham. Yours is the purest form of unconditional love. It is rare and beautiful. Your loss is devastating. It is cruel and unfair. You were both warriors for Graham in life, looking at adversity in the face, laughing and forging on. Dealing with the loss of my beloved dad, I learned that death can only be greeted with acceptance. Even the strongest, the bravest, the purest of heart, must bow to it and accept it without choice. It is the harshest of realities. There are no words to alleviate this pain. I hope that the magical signs you continue to receive, the lifetime of precious memories and the gigantic ripple effect of Graham's life will help sustain you as the days go on. — Kristin O.

ACKNOWLEDGMENTS & CREDITS

Many people helped in the creation of this book. It would have been impossible to write it without the enthusiastic support of Cynthia Gardner. Graham's mom supplied ideas for stories and added important details that had eluded me. Theodore and Deb Lee kindly provided me with the perfect environment for writing. Erik Sayce guided me through the intimidating process of making friends with technology and made significant creative contributions to the project. Paul DeAngeles, Lori Tremblay, Gina Higgins and Anne Richter helped greatly with editing. I am deeply indebted to these individuals. For their friendship and love, I thank my dear friends and all the people of Camp Jabberwocky. To them, I can only say: "O frabjous day! Callooh! Callay! I chortle in my joy."

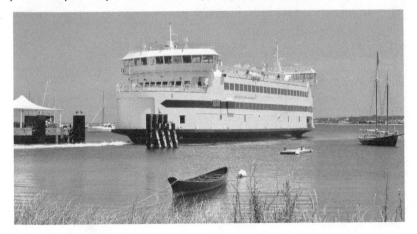

PHOTOS

All photographs by Steven Gardner, except:
Cynthia Gardner: back flap and pp: 6, 80, 97, 115
Lisa Previte: pp: 73, 79, 103, 124, 176, 264
Michael Challik: p. 86
Sidney Morris pp: 35, 192

CONTACTS

Camp Jabberwocky: campjabberwocky.org
Zeno Mountain Farm: zenomountainfarm.org
Handreach: handreach.org
AccesSportAmerica: accessportamerica.org
Spaulding Hospital: spauldingrehab.org
Crotched Mountain: crotchedmountain.org
Special Olympics: specialolympics.org
Pan Mass challenge: pmc.org
The Goldthwait Reservation: goldthwait.org
Steven Gardner Photography: stevengardnerphotography.com

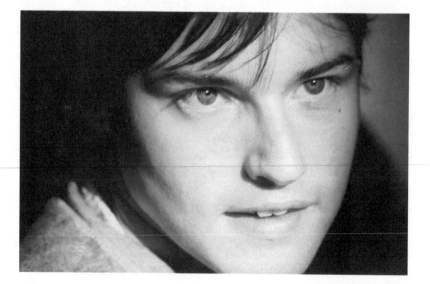